AF564871

Natural Goat Husbandry

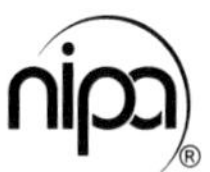

NIPA® GENX ELECTRONIC RESOURCES & SOLUTIONS P. LTD.
New Delhi-110 034

About the Editors

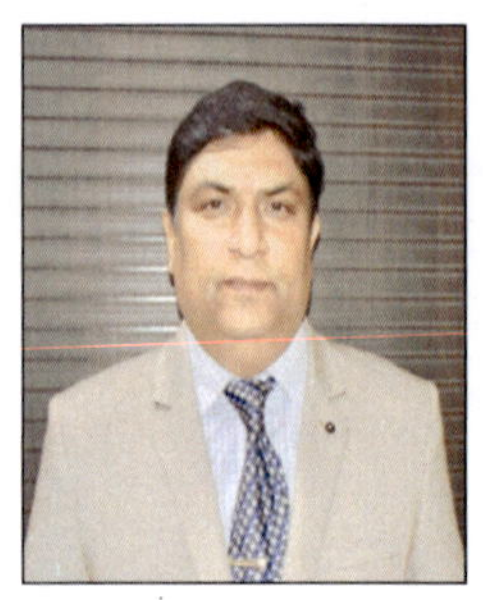

Dr. Ravindra Kumar has completed Bachelor of Veterinary Science and Animal Husbandry from C. V. Sc. & A.H. Mathura with Vice-chancellor University silver medal. He has obtained his M. V. Sc. and Ph.D. degree in Animal Nutrition from ICAR-Indian Veterinary Research Institute, Izatnagar. He was recipient of ICAR (JRF) and IVRI (SRF) during his Master and PhD program respectively. Dr. Kumar has significantly contributed on ruminant nutrition, methane mitigation, unconventional feed utilization, rumen microbiology, complete pellet development, Sulfur hexafluoride technique of methane estimation in goats and rumen microbial culture. During his professional carrier he proved himself as excellent teacher and researcher. He has guided four M.V. Sc. and two Ph. D. students who are well placed. He has handled about twenty two research projects of national interest funded from Department of Biotechnology, Indian council of Agriculture Research, Department of Science and Technology, National Livestock Mission, NABARD etc. He was awarded with International Endeavour Award by Department of Education and Training, Government of Australia. He was on Foreign Deputation at CSIRO, Agriculture and Food, Brisbane, Queensland. He is also recipient of ANA Fellow award, ANA-U.B. Singh Memorial Young Scientist Award 2016, Outstanding achievement award, Best presentation award, ICAR-CIRG appreciation award. He has edited book/ proceedings/newsletters and published around seventy research articles in peer reviewed journals of International/ National repute along with many book chapters and technical articles. He has developed many specialized complete pellet feed, commercialized one technology, two patents and standardized SF6 technique of methane emission in goats. He is life member of many national scientific societies like Animal Nutrition Association, Animal Nutrition society of India, Indian Association for Advancement of Veterinary Research and ISSGPU. He is also the scientific reviewer and editorial Board member of many international like SRR, TAH&P and national scientific Journals.

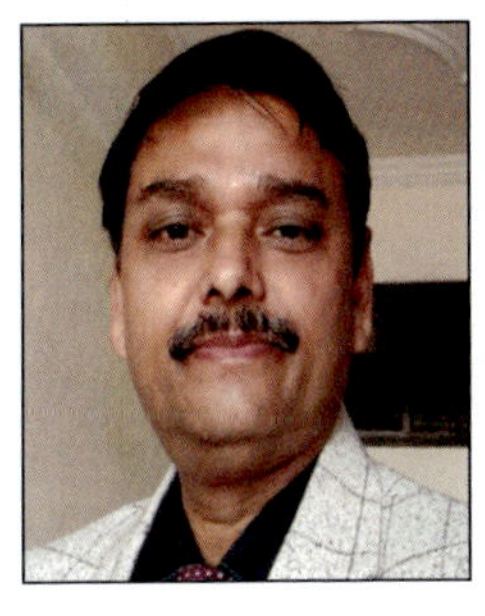

Dr. Anupam Krishna Dixit, currently working as Principal Scientist at the ICAR-Central Institute for Research on Goats, Makhdoom, Mathura. He obtained his MSc in Livestock Economics from ICAR-Indian Veterinary Research Institute (IVRI) and PhD from Institute for Agricultural Sciences (IASc), Banaras Hindu University - BHU. His research interests include Livestock Planning and Development, Environment and Livestock, Agricultural Marketing, Agribusiness Management, and Impact Assessment. Dr. Dixit has published more than 50 research articles in peer-reviewed national and international journals, 4 books, and a discussion paper on International Development Strategies. He has been awarded with Dr. RT Doshi Foundation Award by the Agricultural Economics Research Association, recipient of Best Extension Professional Award from Society of Extension Education. He has been associated with the international project on Environment and Poverty in Urban Informal Sector FASID, Tokyo, Japan and Goat Value Chain project with International Livestock Research Institute (ILRI), Nairobi, Kenya currently, engaged with Department of Science and Technology (DST) project on goat based technological and livelihood improvement in Uttarakhand state and handling NABARD funded project. He has more than 15 years of research experience and worked with Centre for Management in Agriculture (CMA), IIM, Ahmedabad, CESR -NCAP, New Delhi and Sectoral Analysis and Studies Group (SAS), National Dairy Development Board (NDDB), Anand, Gujarat.

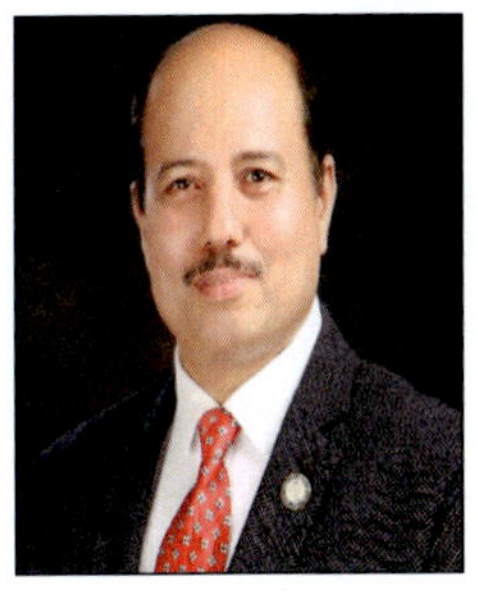

Dr Manish Kumar Chatli has completed his graduation from CCS Haryana Agricultural University and subsequently M VSc in Animal Products Technology, HAU Hisar. Thereafter, he moved to Indian Veterinary Research Institute, Izatnagar for his PhD in Livestock Products Technology. He has gone advance training in proteomics from University of Kentucky, USA. He started his career as Assistant Professor, Department of Livestock Products Technology at CSK HPKV, Palampur. Thereafter, he has been selected as Associate Professor, LPT at PAU/GADVASU. He was promoted to Professor position in 2009 and Head of the department in 2012. He has served HOD, LPT for more than 8 years and HOD, LPM for more than 6 months. He also served as Dean, Ramphura phul, GADVASU, Ludhiana for more than 2 years. He has successfully handled 27 projects from different funding agencies viz. DST, DBT, MoFPI, ICAR,

RKVY, PLDB, NLM etc. He has guided 11 M.V.Sc and 5 PhD students and his 15 PG students received International/National level scholarships/awards/travel grants etc. He has transferred 19 technologies to entrepreneurs. He has established Poultry Processing Plant as Revenue generation Model under Public Private Partnership Mode. He has attended 8 advance trainings/international seminars/workshops in USA, Republic of South Korea, Belgium etc. He has successfully organized 51 trainings, 10 workshop/symposia including International Conference and workshop, ICAR winter course, Entrepreneurship Development Programmes, Model Training Courses, and Industry-Academia-Farmer Interface etc. He has published 2 patents, 8 books, 20 book chapters, 40 manuals/compendiums/research reports and more than 160 research publications in the journal of international & national repute.

Natural Goat Husbandry

Ravindra Kumar
Head and Principal Scientist (Animal Nutrition)
ICAR-CIRG,
Makhdoom, Farah-281122, Uttar Pradesh

A.K. Dixit
Principal Scientist and Head (EE&SE Section)
ICAR-CIRG, Makhdoom
Farah-281122, Mathura, Uttar Pradesh

M.K. Chatli
Director
ICAR-CIRG
Makhdoom, Farah-281122, Uttar Pradesh

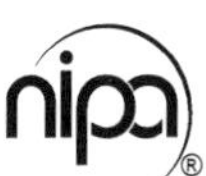

NIPA® GENX ELECTRONIC RESOURCES & SOLUTIONS P. LTD.
New Delhi-110 034

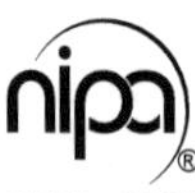

NIPA® GENX ELECTRONIC RESOURCES & SOLUTIONS P. LTD.

NIPA® GENX ELECTRONIC
RESOURCES & SOLUTIONS P. LTD.
101,103, Vikas Surya Plaza, CU Block
L.S.C. Market, Pitam Pura, New Delhi-110 034
Ph : +91-11-43860225, Mob.: +91 9717133558, 9540816132
E-mail: newindiapublishingagency@gmail.com
Website: www.nipaersources.com

Print ISBN: 978-93-5887-807-3

ebook ISBN: 978-93-58874-52-5

Composed and Designed by NIPA®.

Preface

The small ruminant production sector is of great relevance in the world, as sheep and goats represent approximately 56% of the world ruminant population. World herd has approximately 1.2 billion sheep and 1 billion goats growing at around 1.5% per year (FAO, 2016). Small ruminant production plays a crucial socioeconomic role on the different continents. In India as per the latest estimate (20th census) out of total livestock population (536.76 million) the population of goat was 148.88 million representing around 27.74% of total livestock population. In states like West Bengal, Rajasthan and Bihar goat represent 43.50, 36.71 and 35.17% of livestock population. Goat population in India increased from135.17 million (2012) to 148.88 million (2019) representing 10.14% increase in population. Total goat population in rural area has increased by 10.35% whereas in urban area the population of goat has increased by 5.78%. (20th livestock census report, 2019).Goat husbandry practice prevailing in the rural region of India is because of low investment activity. Goats have high fertility and fecundity, low feed and management needs, low investment, high feed conversion efficiency, quick pay-off and low risk involved. The goat sector contributes 8.4 % to the India's livestock GDP. Apart from providing supplementary income to marginal farmers, in recent year's commercial goat farming have emerged as a tool to provide substantial income to progressive farmers in peri-urban region of country. In India mostly small ruminants depend on the diet provided for a small part by rangelands, and mostly by complements, crop residues (cereals, vegetables, etc.) and some forages. The future of the goat industry as a significant economic activity will also be very dependent on the standards of living in the countries where there is a market for goat products. The country is the largest exporter of Sheep & Goat meat to the world. The country has exported 8,695.97 MT of sheep & goat meat to the world for the worth of Rs. 447.58 Crores/ 60.04 USD Millions during the year 2021-22. Utilization and branding of Goat Husbandry as natural practices will further boost the export potential of goat products. In view of the importance of natural goat farming and potential of export of goat products, ICAR-Central Institute for Research on Goat, Makhdoom in collaboration with Agricultural and Processed Food Products Export Development Authority

(APEDA), New Delhi had organized a National level Workshop. This book is the deliberations of the expert in this field. This book will be quite helpful for the goat entrepreneurs, policy makers, researchers and different stakeholder in this area. This will also help to develop strategies and pave a road map for enhancing export of natural goat products to international market.

Editors

Contents

1

Goat Production Under Natural Management System Present Status and Way Forward

A.K. Dixit and Ravindra Kumar

Extension Education and Socio-Economics Section (EE&SE), ICAR-Central Institute for Research on Goats, Makhdoom, Farah, Mathura, Uttar Pradesh

India is home to rich animal resources; it is a source of sustainable livelihood and support during the subsistence crisis of farmers. As per the "First Revised Estimates of National Income, Consumption Expenditure and Capital Formation for 2020-21" released by National Statistical Office (NSO), MoSPI the Gross Value Added (GVA) of livestock sector is about Rs. 11,14,249 crores at current prices during FY 2020-21 which is about 30.87% of Agricultural and Allied Sector GVA and 6.17% of total GVA. At constant prices (2011-12), the GVA of livestock sector is about Rs. 6,17,117 crores during FY 2020-21 with a growth of 6.13% over previous financial year. It contributes about 3.9% to national GDP and 24.8% to agricultural GDP (At 2011-12 Prices) in 2013-14 (GoI 2022). According to the report Situational Assessment of Agricultural Households by the NSSO, a compounded annual income growth rate of 13.7% was observed between 2003 and 2013. Restructuring agriculture processes & policy interventions required to increase the income in real terms (ICFA, 2016). About 29% rural population in the country is below poverty line .Major source of livelihood of rural people is crops, however, it is largely restricted by uncertain and erratic precipitation and low input production system, compelling them for poverty and distress migration. Whereas, small ruminants possess an mechanism for coping up draught because of better adaptability and mobility as compared to crops and large ruminants. Livestock particularly sheep and goat rearing in India is closely interwoven with crop farming. Households cultivating less than 2.0 ha of land (marginal and small) are the main custodian and possess more than 76% goat and 70% of sheep population of the country respectively.

India is home to 148.88 million goats making about 14 percent of the world goat population. Country stood first in goat population, first in goat milk production and second in goat meat and goat skin production in the world. It is an important source of income to farmers particularly in disadvantageous regions in the country where crop failure is the repeated phenomenon. The increasing demand for sheep and goat meat coupled with high conversion efficiency of roughages into protein, milk and meat with other advantages (high prolificacy), short lactation interval and wide range of adaptability, these attributes has made sheep and goat rearing one of preferred and profitable venture. However, actual productivity from these animals is much less than their potential due to poor adoption of critical management practices and inadequate support services.

The demand for goat is basically a derived demand necessitated by the demand for meat, milk, wool, hides, skins etc. High income elastic for livestock products, increasing domestic consumption due to increment in per capita income growth, variation in taste preference urbanization and increasing nutrition literacy are some of the driving factors of increasing demand for livestock products.Globally the demand for livestock products, particularly for chevon and mutton is on rise, due to the increase in per capita income in developing countries.In the present paper, an attempt was made to explore the importance of goat sector, socio-economic status of goat farmers, goat production under natural management system and its export potential The inferences drawn from present analysis on country's goat production — would help in planning to formulate natural resource based goat development programmes.

Goat Sector: Present status and Opportunities

India is home to 149 million goats making about 14 percent of the world goat population. Country has 37 descript breeds of goats. Goat sector contributes about 8% to the total value of output (at current prices) from livestock sector. Ownership pattern of goats among different land holding categories indicated that more than 75% goats have been reared by the marginal and small holdings. It showed the importance of goat among resource poor people for their sustainable livelihood and nutritional requirement. The gap between demand and supply of goat meat /mutton will widen in future as meat demand may grow at faster rate than that of production. Goat milk which is also known as natural functional food contributes 3% to central milk pool (210 million tonnes). Majority of goats in the country are reared under extensive production system and highly depended on common resources. Permanent pasture and grazing lands which is one of the most important commons is gradually shrinking (Dixit et al 2015).

Dominance of Small Holders

Goat value chain is basically small holders' goat value chain, more than 73% of goats are possessed by the marginal and small landholdings. The share of goat ownership has improved with marginal category by 2% between 2001-02 and 2006-07. Small and marginal together constitute about 83% of total land holdings. This indicates that the importance of small ruminants is continuing to be strong as a livelihood support to resource poor households. Moreover, goats are inclusively distributed among other species of ruminants. The preference for smaller animals (sheep, goat and poultry) is stronger towards the lower-end of land distribution. This is because of low investment and higher returns due to shorter gestation periods and higher prolificacy rates (Jumrani & Birthal 2015).

Goats and Livestock Economy

Small ruminant sector contributes about 12% to national economy. Goat which is known as poor man's cow has now becoming a symbol of prosperity in rural India. The rural poor who cannot afford large ruminants, find goat as the best alternative for supplementary income and milk. Demographic change in livestock population in the country showed a shift in favor of small ruminant particularly for goat (Dikshit et al., 2012). Moreover, goat has a tremendous potential to adapt in different agro-climatic conditions and on wide range of feedings. The goats and its products contribute Rs. 38,590 crore annually to the national economy. This accounts for 8.4% to total value of output (at current prices) from livestock sector in 2010-11. Goat meat alone contributes about Rs. 22625 crores (59%) to total value of output from goat sector followed by milk (Rs.9564 crores), by-products (Rs.3005 crores), manure (Rs.1535 crores). Despite of its significant contribution to the livestock economy, the sector could not receive attention as it deserves.

Population Dynamics

There is significant growth in population of goat in India during the last three decades. As per 20th livestock census 2019, goat population in India has increased from 135 to 149 million between and 2012 (Table-1). The highest increase in goat population (16%) was recorded during 1982 to 1987. About 13% increase has been recorded between 2007 and 2003 and recorded 10% between 2012 and 2019. Growth in goat population is demand- driven. In urban areas, demand for livestock products rises faster than the other food groups when income starts to increase. Compound annual growth has been worked out for different sets of census periods (Table-4). Annual growth in goat population was recorded about 3 per cent during 1982 to 1987. However, it has declined to 0.27% during 1997 to 2003 but further increase and maintained about 2.5% during 2003 to 2007. The growth between 2007 and 2012 was found negative as goat population has gone down by 5 million between the same periods. However, again maintained to 1.38% between 2012 and 2019.

Table 1: Trends in Goat Population

Census year	Goat Population (million)	Periods	% increase/ decrease	CAGR (%)
1982	95	-	-	-
1987	110	1987-82	15.79	2.96
1992	115	1992-87	4.55	0.90
1997	123	1997-92	6.45	1.26
2003	124	2003-97	1.34	0.27
2007	140	2007-03	13.01	2.48
2012	135	2012-07	-3.82	-0.78
2019	149	2012-19	10.37	1.38

Adoption of improved management practices will increase population growth by cutting down mortality among kids and adults and productivity. Major impediment in increasing the small ruminants' population is the dwindling area and productivity of pastures.Shrinking pastures and grazing lands is more concern to goat keepers because majority of them are resource poor and largely dependent on such resources for grazing and gleaning grasses. Analysis indicated that the decline in total goat population between 2007 and 2012 was due to decline in all the categories of male goats including breeding bucks. However, growth in recent past indicated that goat farming in the country gaining momentum. Large number of goat farms under semi-intensive and intensive management have started production in different parts of the country.

Production Performance of Goats: Meat and Milk

Small ruminants together constitute 24% of total meat production. Goat meat (Chevon) is a main staple red meat in human diets without any social restrictions. Goats are an important nutrient (protein) source in the world, particularly for people situated mainly in the tropics. The distribution of goat population in the world comprises with approximately 51% in Asia, 43% in Africa and 4.0% in America, Oceana and the Caribbean (FAOSTAT, 2020). Goat contributes 13 per cent to country's total meat production however, poultry is having lion share (36%) to the total meat production from all the species (fig-1). Goat meat production increased from 0.398 to 1.21 million tons between 2003-04 and 2020-21 (Table-2). However, meat yield increased from 9.64 to 10.74 kg/animal during 2003 to 2013.

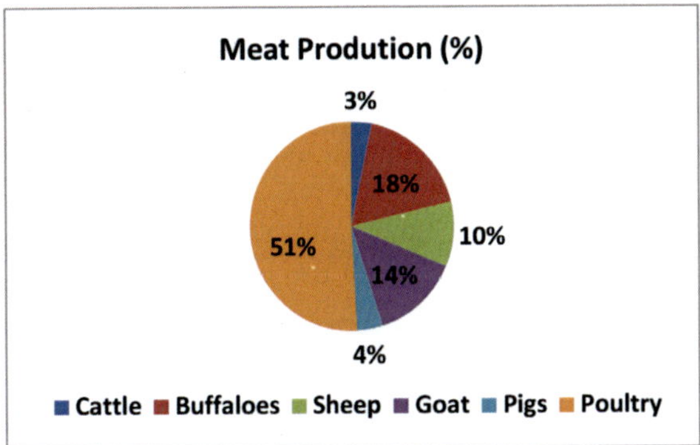

Sheep meat (Mutton) production in the country has increased from 0.60 million tonnes to 0.88 million tones between 2017-18 and 2020-21. The average carcass yield was estimated to be 13.5 kg in the year 2020-21.

Similarly, goat milk production almost doubled between 2003-04 and 2020-21. It has increased from 3.7 million tonnes in 2003-04 to 6.26 million tonnes in 2020-21. However, milk yield has increased only by hardly 150 grams/animal between the same period. The impressive growth in meat production in the country resulted mainly due to increase in number of animals slaughtered. Productivity of goat for meat and milk is low and attributed mainly to poor adoption of technologies.

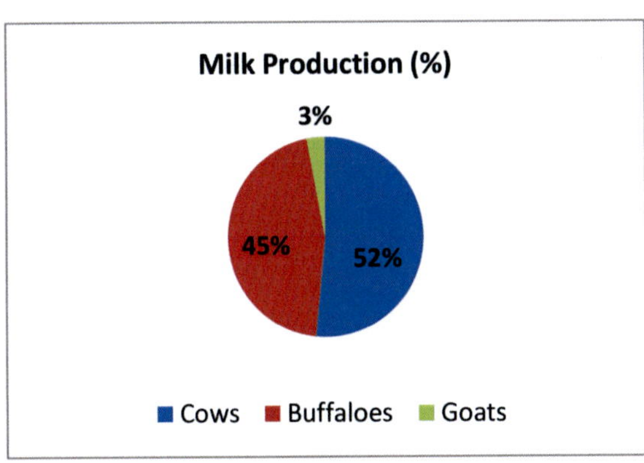

Table 2: Trends in Goat Milk and Meat Production in India

Year	Goat Milk Production (million tonnes)	Goat Meat Production (million tonnes)	Milk yield (kg/animal)	Meat yield (kg/animal)
2003-04	3.71	0.398	0.314	9.64
2007-08	4.48	0.488	0.390	11.00
2012-13	5.05	0.941	0.430	10.74
2020-21	6.26	1.21	0.470	11.36

Source: Basic Animal Husbandry Statistics (various issues)

Contribution of Goat Rearing in Present Household Income

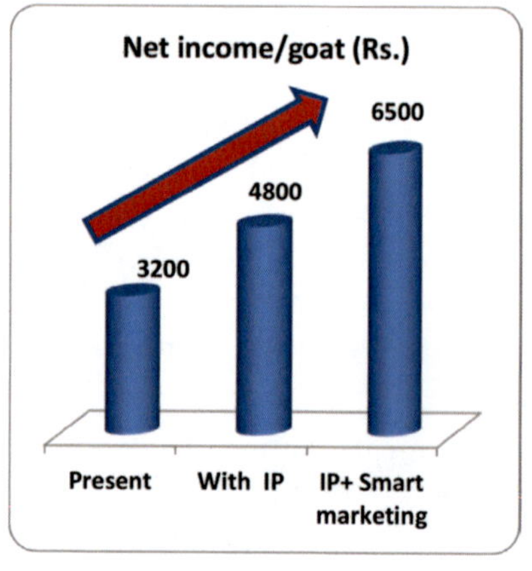

More than 75% goats are reared by marginal and small households under extensive management system. Studies revealed that in general, goat rearing contributes about 15% to the total household income of goat farmers and generates gainful employment to rural farm families. However, out of 135.04 million goats, 26.97% are pure bred, 11.77% are graded breeds and remaining 61.26% are non- descript. Field studies indicated that net income per goat per year was about Rs.3200.00, by and large low in productivity and fetch less price. With some little input on nutrition, health and management, the income per adult goat per year was improved to Rs. 4800.00 (1.5 times). Goat farmers rearing goats under semi-intensive /intensive management system and with smart marketing may earn profit at the tune of Rs. 6500.00 per adult goat per year (double of extensive management system). By doubling income per goat per year, the contribution of goat rearing to the household's income may increase from 15 to 30%. It needs effective support services (prophylactic) from state animal husbandry department, micro credit facilities from financial institutions for increased adoption of technologies and setting up of commercial goat farms, market and cooperative departments.

Goat which is known as poor man's cow has now becoming a symbol of prosperity in rural India. Goat rearing plays an important role in livelihood security of millions of landless, marginal and small farmers. Starting of dairy farm with cows and buffaloes has become an expensive business as it requires high capital cost in the beginning. Therefore, goat farming is now preferred small scale business among resource poor farmers. A farmer initiate goat rearing with 50 goats of Barbari breed require a capital of about Rs.6-7 lakh. Goat rearing at small scale may utilize family labour (women labour) efficiently and the problem of malnutrition in women and children may also solved. An economic analysis of goat unit with 50 does and 2 male bucks of Barbari breed is given below:

Economic analysis of goat unit of 50+2

A. Expenditure (Rs.)

a. Capital cost

(i) Goat shed	1,25,000.00
(ii) Equipment	20,000.00
(iii) 50 Barbari goats @ Rs.6000/- per goat (pregnant)	3,00,000.00
(iv) 2 Breeding buck @ Rs.8000/- per buck	16,000.00
Total capital cost	4,61,000.00

b. Recurring cost

(i) Feed cost (concentrate feed) Adult does, bucks and kids (@ 250-300 gram per adult goat & kid per day for 200-220 days)	1,08,540.00
(ii) Health management cost (@Rs.80/animal/year)	10,560.00
(iii) Labour (imputed value of grazing) @ Rs.4000/month	48,000.00
Total recurring cost	1,67,100.00
Gross cost	6,28,100.00

B. Income (Rs.)

(i) Sale of kids (76 kids of 20-22 kg body weight at 9-10 month @ Rs.250/kg/live weight)	4,18,000.00
(ii) Value of 52 adult goats at the end of year	3,31800.00
(iii) Depreciated value of shed (@10% per year)	1,10,500.00
(iv) Sale of milk (after feeding kids)	21,600.00
(v) Value of goat manure and others	10,000.00
Total income	8,91,900.00
Net income	2,63,800.00
Net income per month	21,983.00
Net return per doe	5,276.00

It is clear from economic analysis that if a poor farmer start goat rearing with a unit of 50 goats and adopt scientific practices, he may earn net income about Rs.2,64,000.00 annually. Per goat per year net income would be about Rs.5300.

Goat Based Integrated Livelihood Models for Rain-Fed/ Disadvantageous Regions

Livelihood models for different categories (resources) farmers were suggested based on implemented interventions among goat farmers in Bundelkhand region of Uttar Pradesh (Table-3). Model revealed that a landless /marginal household having 15 adult female goats and 25 poultry birds may yield Rs. 82727 per annum. Similarly, a landless/marginal/small household with 10 adult goats, 2 cows and 50 chicks and 1 ha rain-fed land may earn Rs. 100634 per year. Marginal, small and medium farmers with 5 adult female goats, 2 buffalo, 2 cows and 2 ha of rain-fed land may earn Rs. 119000 per year. Whereas, a semi-medium, medium and large farmer may earn Rs. 119000 per year with keeping 10 goats, 2 buffaloes, 2 cows and crop production on 2 ha semi-irrigated land. These recommended models were highly adopted among farmers as they were developed through participatory research with farmers.

Table 3: Goat based Integrated Livelihood Models

S.No	Model	Unit	Net income (Rs)	Suitability for household category	Number of HH Covered under trial
1	Goat+	15 adult F+	Rs 82727	Landless	64
	Poultry	25 Chicks	(71115+11612)	Marginal	
2	Goat+	10 adult F+	Rs 100634	Landless	142
	Cow+	2 cows +	(47410+22000+ 23224+8000)	Marginal	
	Poultry+	50 chicks +		Small	
	Crops (Rain-fed)	1 ha.			
3	Goat+	5 adult F +	Rs 109705	Marginal	80
	Buffaloes+	2 buffaloes+	(23705+34000+	Small	
	Cows+	2 cows +	22000+30000	Medium large	
	Crop (semi-irri)	2 ha.			
4	Goat	10 adult F	Rs 119000	Semi-medium	56
	Buffaloes	2 buffaloes	(47410+32000+	Medium	
	Cows	2 cows	22000+30000)	Large	
	Crop (semi-irri)	2 ha			

Source: Singh et al. 2013

Goat Production under Natural Management System

The basic motive behind natural farming is to discourage chemicals and other externally purchased input use and move towards traditional farming method. It is considered as agro-ecology based diversified farming system which develop synergism with crops, trees and livestock with functional biodiversity.

In India, Natural farming is promoted as Bharatiya Prakritik Krishi Paddhati Programme (BPKP) under centrally sponsored scheme- Paramparagat Krishi Vikas Yojana (PKVY). BPKP is aimed at promoting traditional indigenous practices which reduces externally purchased inputs. It is largely based on on-farm biomass recycling with major stress on biomass mulching, use of on-farm cow dung-urine formulations; periodic soil aeration and exclusion of all synthetic chemical inputs. It is roughly estimated that around 2.5 million farmers in India are already practicing regenerative agriculture. In the next 5 years, it is expected to reach 20 lakh hectares- in any form of organic farming, including natural farming, of which 12 lakh hectares are under BPKP.

According to HLPE Report (The **High Level Panel of Experts on Food Security and Nutrition** of the Committee on World Food Security (CFS) is the United Nations body for assessing the science related to world food security and nutrition), natural farming will reduce dependency on purchased inputs and will help to ease smallholder farmers from credits burden (www.niti.gov.in). It provides **independent, comprehensive and evidence-based analysis,** and elaborates its studies through a scientific, **transparent and inclusive process**.

By virtue of its simplicity, majority of goat are reared under extensive management system- close to natural production system. However, the research on natural livestock production has not got momentum so far. There is need to document traditional practices such as local resource based feed options, use of locally available material for low cost housing, climate resilient feed fodder options, use of animal waste as manure and develop training modules for value addition of goat milk and meat based products and enabling environment for export promotion.

Major Constraints Goat Production under Natural Management System

In spiteof having potential of good economic returns from small ruminant rearing, goat farmers havevery poor income levels. There may be a number of reasons for it and summarized briefly as follows:

i. Scarcity of superior bucks-Breed dilution is common feature due to indiscriminate breeding. Sale of males with higher growth rate at 3-6 months of age and small flock holders are not willing to keep breeding buck, thus low potential males are being used for breeding the goats. The availability of purebred breed bucks of high genetic merit is very –very low (1:80-100 does) in sheep and goatkeepers flock.

ii. Knowledge gap on natural resource based scientific interventions and technologies have not yet been effectively disseminated and adopted by the goat keepers.

iii. Scarcity of feed and fodder: Under feeding and inadequate housing further deteriorate the immunity level of animals and made them vulnerable for diseases. During last few decades' sheep and goat flock and herd sizes were reducing due to shrinkage of common grazing resources and deficiency of biomass in rangelands.

iv. Higher mortality on account of very low adoption of prophylactic and curative health measures: Prophylactic health measures were highly uncertain and followed by few farmers. Lack of knowledge on ethno veterinary based solutions.

v. Inadequate housing- goats were housed predominately in human dwelling, in open and under enclosures made up bush and shrubs.

vi. Depletion of grazing resources due to over grazing on account of very high stocking rate and poor management of grazing resources.Expenditure on feed and fodder account for more than 60% of recurring cost, which matter for landless goat and sheep keepers and small land holders. During draught or flood the availability of biomass from CPR reduces from 3.5 q/ha to 0.5 q/ha per year. Thus productivity, survivability and income go down upto70%.

vii. Low availability of veterinary and other support services mainly institutional credit to goat keepers.

viii. Low price realization due to unorganized marketing and lack of milk cooperatives.Majority of small ruminants was sold through middlemen and share of middle man in total income varied from 15-35%. Distress sale of goat due to very urgent natures of domestic needs and thus farmers realized lesser share of income.

ix. Lack of infrastructure on value addition and knowledge to link export linked commercial venture.

Recommendations

1. Development of genetic stock by supply of high potential pure-bred bucks to farmers.
2. Grading up of non-descript goats/poor performance goats with pure bred bucks of high genetic merit suitable for that particular agro-climatic regions.
3. Encourage natural resource based low cost interventions.

4. Development of forage resources in community land.
5. Promotion of herbal based prophylactic measures which include proper vaccination and deworming.
6. Clean and adequate housing as per breed, age, sex and production stage.
7. Value addition of goat products and by products.
8. Popularization of natural resource based economic viable models suitable for different regions.
9. Support for regulatory market of goat and credit support to poor goat farmers and linking them export oriented units.
10. Capacity building of goat farmers on improved practices.

References

Birthal P S and Taneja V K.2006. Livestock sector in India:Opportunities and challenges for small holders In: Proceedingsof an ICAR-ILRI International Workshop, NCAP, New Delhi and ILRI, Nairobi.

Dikshit,A.K., Reddy,B.S., and Manohar,N.S., 2012. Demographic changes in small ruminant population in India: Some inferences from different livestock regions. Indian Journal of Animal Sciences 82 (2): 187–193, February 2012

Dixit, A.K., Singh M.K. and Gopal Das 2018. Small ruminant farming and livelihood security in India: Present status and opportunities for enhancing farmers' income (DOI: 10.5958/2394-4471.2017.00043.0). International Conference Special Issue on Sustainability of Smallholder Agriculture under Changing Climatic Scenario organised by the Society of Agricultural Professionals, Chandra Shekhar Azad University of Agriculture & Technology Kanpur. February 14-17, 2018.

Dixit A.K., Singh, M.K., Roy,A.K., Reddy B.S. and Singh, N. 2015 Trends and contribution of grazing resources to livestock in different states of India. Range Management and Agroforestry. Vol. 36, Issue 2 pp. 204-210.

Dixit A.K. and Mohan Braj. (2014). Economics of goat production in Mathura district of Uttar Pradesh. The Indian Journal of Small Ruminants 20(2): 96-98.

Dixit A.K. and Singh M.K. (2014). Economic analysis of goat rearing under field conditions of Bundelkhand Region. The Indian Journal of Small Ruminants 20 (2): 165-168.

Dixit A.K. and Singh M.K. (2014). Factors determining flock size of goats in Bundelkhand region of Uttar Pradesh. Agricultural Economics Research Review. 27 (2): 315-318.

Dixit A K, Birthal P S and Bhatt A B.Role of credit in goat marketing, Agricultural Marketing Vol.XXVII, No. 3.1995.

Dixit A K, Mohan Braj, Singh K and Kumar Vijay. (2014). Impact of training programme on goat farmers and stakeholders: A study of CIRG training programmes. Indian Research Journal of Extension Education 14 (3):112-114.

Dixit A K, Singh S K, Tripathi M K, Singh M K and Kumar Vijay. 2015.Economic Gains from Technological and Market Interventions in Goat Production in India. An Ex-ante Assessment. Agricultural Economics Research Review28 (2):285-292.

Gandhi, Vasant P and Zhou,Zhy-Yue, 2010. Rising demand for livestock products in India:Nature,pattern and implications. Australian Agribusiness Review, Vol.18, Paper 7, ISSN 1442-6951.

Government of India 2005.18th Livestock Census, 2007. Deaprtment of Animal Husbandry and Dairying, New Delhi.Government of India 2012, Basic Animal Husbandry Statistics, Department of Animal Husbandry and Dairying (www.dahd.nic.in).

Government of India 2013.Key Indicators of Situation of Agricultural Households in India. 70th Round (Jan- December 2013). Ministry of Statistics and Programme Implementation, National Sample Survey Office, New Delhi.

Indian Council of Food and Agriculture, 2016. Report on Doubling Farmer's Income by 2022 Farm Crisis and Farmers' Distress. India International Centre, New Delhi

Jumrani J. and Birthal P.S. 2015. Livestock, Women, and Child Nutrition in Rural India Agricultural Economics Research Review Vol. 28 (No.2) July-December 2015 pp 223-246

Pasha, S M., 2000.Economy and ecological dimensions of livestock economy.Commonwealth publishers, New Delhi.

Pollot G. and Wilson R.T., 2009, Sheep and Goats for diverse products and profits (FAO Rome).

Rai B, Singh M K and Singh S K. 2005. Goats for meat, milk and fiber: A Review: Indian Journal of Animal Sciences. 75 (3):335-349.

Singh M K, Dixit A K, Roy A K and Singh S K. 2014.Analysis of Prospects and Problems of Goat Production in Bundelkhand Region.Range Management and Agro-forestry: 35(1):163-168.

Singh M K, Dixit A K, RoyA K and Singh S K 2013. Goat Rearing: A Pathway for Sustainable Livelihood Security in Bundelkhand Region: Agricultural Economics Research Review26:79-88.

Singh M K, Goel A K, Rai B, Kumar Ashok and SharmaM C. 2010. Impact of breed improvement programme on goat production under farmers' flocks Indian Journal of Animal Sciences 80 (4): 379–38.

Singh M K, Rai B, Singh Pallavi, Singh P K, and Singh N P. 2008. Status of goat production in different agro-climatic regions of India.An Overview. Indian Journal of Small Ruminants 14(1) 48-70.

Singh M K and Dixit A K.2016.Improving Livelihood of Rural Population through Goat Farming in India: Prospects and Potential.Book on "Conservation of Indigenous Domestic Animal Biodiversity" Published by NBAGR, Karnal. ISBN: 978-93-83537-29-7 : Page No 148-162.

Singh M Kand Singh S K. 2015.Goat Genetic Resources of India: Strategies for their Improvement and Conservation. International Symposium on" Sustainable Management of Animal Genetic Resources for Livelihood Security in Developing Countries". Society for Conservation of Domestic Animal Biodiversity (SOCDAB): 13-14 Feb, 2015, TANUVASU Chennai in collaboration with Animal Convention of Society forConservation of Domestic Animal Biodiversity (SOCDAB). Published in Compendium. Page No - 109-116

2

Organic Livestock Rearing Opportunity for Export & Domestic Market

Mahesh Chander

Division of Extension Education ICAR- Indian Veterinary Research Institute Izatnagar, Uttar Pradesh

Organic Animal Husbandry happens to be an emerging area which requires attention given its growing potential for domestic as well as export market. The start-ups including farmers engaged in organic farming and entrepreneurs need support in terms of information, technical knowledge, financial, incubation, hand-holding and marketing of organic animal products. Organic animal husbandry has been defined as a system of livestock production that promotes the use of organic and biodegradable inputs from the ecosystem deliberately avoiding the use of synthetic inputs such as drugs, feed additives and genetically engineered breeding inputs, while ensuring the welfare of animals. There are four principles of organic farming viz; principle of ecology, principle of health, principle of fairness, and principle of care, which organic systems must always take into consideration. In order to achieve the animal welfare, environmental protection, resource-use sustainability and other objectives, certain key principles are adhered to under organic livestock production systems. The organic livestock & poultry standards have been notified by APEDA under National Programme for Organic Production (NPOP). All operations related to organic livestock including goat & poultry production are to be governed by these standards in India.

The start-ups, including farmers engaged in organic farming and entrepreneurs, need support in terms of information, technical knowledge, finances, incubation and marketing of organic animal products. The extension and advisory services institutions have to provide prompt technical know-how and impart skills to field extension workers and farmers. For this, emphasis has to be given to start-up programmes that transform aspiring farmers into agripreneurs of organic animal husbandry. People all over the world are becoming increasingly aware and conscious about the naturally available products and their importance in their daily life. The Indian consumers are increasingly looking for safe, unadulterated, healthy foods including organic labeled milk. If not for self initially, but surely for their kids to begin with, where milk is part and parcel of their daily food. So it is the Indian dairy farmer, who has to en-cash the emerging situation and consider to switch over to organic livestock farming. Thus, demand for information on how to do organic farming is increasing at the level of farmers. It's a highly knowledge and skill based system of production, so farmers have to acquire a lot of information and learn skills from the right sources in order to become a successful organic dairy farmer.

The National Programme on Organic Production (NPOP) & Organic Livestock Production

The Agricultural and Processed Food Products Export Development Authority (APEDA) implements India's National Programme on Organic Production (NPOP). Out of 32 accredited certification bodies (CBs) in India currently, 7 CBs are accredited by APEDA for certification of livestock and poultry. Also, it has taken initiatives to train certification bodies and evaluation committee to inspect and audit organic livestock operations. The APEDA has been organizing capacity-building programmes for inspectors/auditors on organic livestock certification process towards developing organic animal husbandry in India. The start-ups wishing to convert to organic animal husbandry need to be aware of organic livestock production's conversion, production and certification procedures (NPOP, 2015).

To be a successful organic livestock farmer, the following traits are expected from a farmer

- Willing to learn and take risk, in new ventures likes organic livestock farming.
- Owning land good enough to raise number of animals as per the carrying capacity, wherein, livestock can be housed and maintained as per prescribed space requirements, fodder could be grown and also animals let loose for grazing and exercise, at least for a few hours in a day.
- She considers that organic livestock farming can be done sustainably under integrated crop-livestock production systems.
- If a farmer is literate, can read and write, it would help him/her follow the literature on organic farming, leaflets, folders, manuals etc.
- Willingness to participate in training programmes on agricultural development issues including organic farming.

- Having an interest in diversifying the farm activities by including more crops, number of livestock species etc. on farm.
- A willing person to not to inflict cruelty on animals and ever ready for adoption of animal welfare practices. S/he gives humane treatment to animals, keeps animals and their dwellings clean, comfortable and germ free and avoids taking work from sick and injured animals. S/he does not discriminate or neglect old and infertile animals at his/her farm.
- S/he maintains written records of farm activities, making available the records of inputs used, breeding records, treatment details, feeding schedules, whenever asked.
- A farmer who updates himself about latest Good Agricultural Practices and other similar aspects towards ensuring quality of agricultural products.
- S/he ensures that his children attend schools and does not employ his minor children in agricultural activities at the expense of their educational activities as far as possible.
- S/he does not discriminate between male and female laborers in matters of wages and other benefits.
- S/he largely avoids taking services of quacks for treatment of animals, but actively seeks professionally qualified veterinary health care whenever animals face health problems.
- S/he tries to exploit on farm resources as far as possible, reducing his/her reliance on market purchased inputs.
- S/he prefers to minimizing the use of fossil fuel driven machines.
- S/he grows green fodder for livestock using available on farm resources to the extent possible. S/he offers animals' clean and organically grown fodder and feeds.
- S/he tries to seek professional assistance to raise his/her livestock as per the prescribed norms through suitable agencies (government, private sector, NGOs, cooperatives).
- S/he promotes indigenous breeds, prefers local but safe and valid practices of health management, and encourages the practice of dry dairy.
- S/he does not use chemical fertilizers/agrochemicals on his/her farm. S/he doesn't burn crop residues and other agro wastes, but actively promote scientific animal waste management practices like, composting, biogas, vermi-composting and making bio-fertilizers and biomaterials from cow

dung and cattle urine for improving soil fertility and controlling pests and disease of crops.

- S/he follows crop rotations, prefers leguminous crops, and tries to minimize practices which increases pollution.
- Ideally, S/he is concerned for environment, ecology, soil, human and animal health, thus, exercise caution, implements safety measures on his/her farm, follow a healthy lifestyle, takes good care of people and animals around him/her.

Organic Animal Husbandry: The Key Considerations

The major challenge in organic livestock production systems is to honour the organic principles in a wide range of diverse systems under a wide range of circumstances and conditions including systems which are not yet certified 'organic' at the moment. It's recommended that developing organic animal husbandry at all times require a thorough analysis of the problems, opportunities and existing local knowledge. Therefore, some key considerations in organic animal husbandry that producers and other stakeholders need to take into account are listed here under:

***Origin of Livestock*:** Livestock and products from the livestock that are sold, labeled, or advertised as organic must be from livestock that originate from animals that were managed under continuous organic management from the last third of gestation or at hatching.

***Livestock Feed*:** Livestock that are produced under organic management must have their total ration that is comprised of agricultural products including pasture, forage, and crops that are organically produced and handled organically. There are certain non-synthetic and synthetic substances that can be used as feed additives and supplements. Dairy cattle under 9 months of age are allowed 20% of their feed coming from non-organic sources. Plastic pellets, urea, manure, mammalian or poultry slaughter by-products are not allowed. The list of allowed and non allowed feeding material is available as annexures with the organic livestock and poultry standards developed among others by Government of India.

***Living Conditions*:** An organic livestock producer must create and maintain living conditions that accommodate natural behavior and health of the animal. The living conditions must include access to outdoors, shade, shelter, fresh air, direct sunlight suitable to the species, and access to pasture for ruminants.

***Waste Management*:** Organic livestock producers are mandated to manage manure so that it does not contribute to the contamination of crops, soil, or water and optimizes recycling of nutrients.

Health Care: Organic livestock production practices require the producer to establish preventative health care practices. The health care practices include selecting the appropriate species and type of livestock, providing adequate feed, create an appropriate environment that minimizes stress, disease, parasites, administration of vaccines and veterinary biologics and animal husbandry practices to promote animal wellbeing in a manner that minimizes pain and stress. Producers cannot provide preventative antibiotics. Producers are encouraged to treat animals with appropriate treatment, including antibiotics and other conventional medicines when needed but treated animals can not be sold or labeled as organic. Producers can not administer hormones or other drugs for growth promotion.

***Record Keeping/Audit Trail*:** Organic livestock operations need to maintain records for a number of reasons. Apart from financial management of the organic livestock enterprise, records are important for the verification of organic status of animals, production, harvesting, and handling practices associated with the organic products and animals. Records are mandated to be maintained for 5 years, and must demonstrate compliance with the organic food production standards and acts, if any in place.

Under organic livestock production systems, it is expected that- organic milk, meat, poultry, eggs and products thereof come from farms that have been inspected to verify that they meet rigorous standards which mandate the use of organic feed, prohibit the use of antibiotics, give animals' access to outdoor, fresh air and sunlight. The production methods are selected based on criteria that meet all health regulations, work in harmony with the environment, build biological diversity and foster healthy soil and growing conditions. After the production, animals are marketed that were raised without use of toxic persistent pesticides, antibiotics and paraciticides. Animal health, well being, better living conditions, welfare measures, feeding practices are to be ensured through a set of standards and maintenance of written records by the organic livestock farmers. Better managemental practices and prevention are emphasized over treatment. Thus, the primary characteristics of organic livestock production system are: a defined standard; greater attention to animal welfare; no routine use of growth promoters, animal offal or any other additives; at least 80% of feed grown according to organic standards, without the use of artificial fertilizers or pesticides on the crops or grass. To be precise, organic meat, milk and eggs means that are produced, harvested, preserved and processed as per organic standards. Anyone wishing to switch over or convert to organic farming need to follow the organic standards developed among others by Government of India under National Programme for Organic Production (NPOP, 2024).

Organic production systems are knowledge and skill intensive, where the producers are expected to be knowledgeable about production norms, standards and practices for production and processing prescribed under approved standards by the designated authorities viz APEDA, BIS, FSSAI etc. It is expected from the organic producers that they are not only familiar with organic livestock standards, but also well versed in good agricultural/livestock production practices, animal welfare standards, regulatory requirements as applicable to livestock and food production in general. At one end, there is traditional animal husbandry, while conventional production system in between and the most innovative one i.e. organic animal husbandry is the latest system. The farmers wishing to switch from traditional and conventional animal production systems to organic animal husbandry need information, knowledge and skills to follow organic livestock and poultry standards, where there exists currently a big gap. Field level extension functionaries need to have wider awareness and knowledge about organic animal husbandry standards for onward dissemination of information and orientation of the stakeholders involved in livestock production.

The organic livestock development opportunities in developing countries in Asia, Africa and Latin America can be enhanced with more scientific research in organic livestock/poultry production under local conditions and strengthening institutional support. Organic agriculture is rapidly growing around the world including in India (Table1).

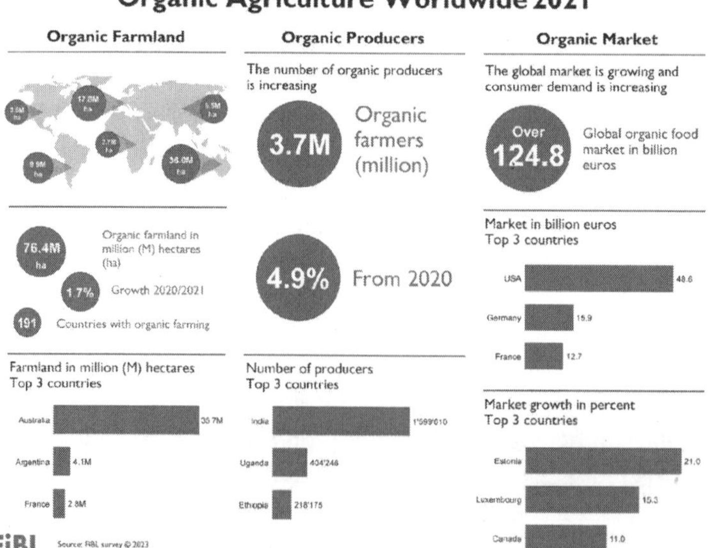

Table1: Organic: The global scenario

- Over 4.43 Million producers grow organic foods in 99 Million ha land across 188 countries resulting in 136 billion Euro global market for organic products. (Willer, Trávníček and Schlatter, 2025).
- Organic milk production currently stands at 4.4million metric tons (European Union: 4.1 million), constituting more than 2.8 percent of the European Union's milk production from dairy cows in 2016
- As per USDA, sales of organic broilers in US in 2017 rose by 78% to $750m, making it the largest growing market in the organic sector, while organic egg sales rose by 11% to $816m

India: An organic Success Story

- With 1.6 Million producers India continues to be No. 1 country
- India ranks 2nd in terms of area & 1st in terms of number of certified organic producers
- 4.43 million organic farmers, and about 5.91 Million ha area has been brought under organic farming by 2021-22 (Economic Survey 2022-23)
- Sikkim with 58,168 ha under organic farming is 1st state in the world to become fully organic
- India exported 460320.40 MT organic products worth US$771.96 million during 2021-22
- GoI is promoting organic and natural farming through various schemes of *Paramparagat Krishi Vikas Yojana* (PKVY), since 2014
- Under PKVY, as of 16 November 2022, 32,384 clusters totalling 0.64 million ha area and 1.61 million farmers have been covered
- The National Mission for Clean Ganga (NMCG) or "*Namami Gange*" has initiated a project for promoting organic farming in the villages situated along the river
- Under *Namami Gange* Programme, 0.12 Million ha area has been covered under organic farming
- Government support to Organic Agriculture & Natural Farming
- In the Union budget 2022-23, the Government of India launched National Mission on Natural Farming *(NMNF) by up-scaling the Bharatiya Prakritik Krishi Paddhati* (BPKP) for promotion of natural farming on a bigger scale
- The DAC&FW is conducting large scale training of Master Trainers, Champion Farmers and other farmers on latest methods of Natural Farming with the help of National Institute of Agricultural Extension Management (MANAGE) and National Center of Organic and Natural Farming (NCONF). MANAGE has also imparted training on natural farming to *Gram Pradhans*
- ICAR Institutes including KVKs are conducting training, trials & demonstrations on Natural Farming
- Master's course in Organic Agriculture approved & course curriculum on Natural farming is being developed
- Many FPOs/FPCs, SHGs are engaged in organic production, processing & marketing
- On 1st February, 2023, a new programme "PM PRANAM" has been launched to give further boost to chemical free farming

The Government of India (GOI) has taken several initiatives to boost organic agricultural production in the country. The launching of National Programme of Organic Production (NPOP) in 2000-2001, setting up of National Centre of Organic Farming (NCOF) at Ghaziabad during 2003-04, ICAR Network Project on Organic Farming (2004) are some important milestones. These steps have resulted into significant increase in production and export of certified organic agricultural products from India. Most of the organic agricultural products currently exported from India are of plant origin except honey. Organic Animal products are also showing up in market through slowly. There are 52 certified organic dairy operators, 66 meat operators & 3 certified egg operators in India. The information on domestic sales of organic livestock products indicate the availability of certified organic milk and milk products in India (Table1). Also, India exported 2125.6 kg of certified organic *Ghee* (Clarifed butter) to UAE during 2019-20. Animals not only produce products for direct human consumption, but also help produce organic by-products like cattle urine & cow dung used to enhance soil fertility.

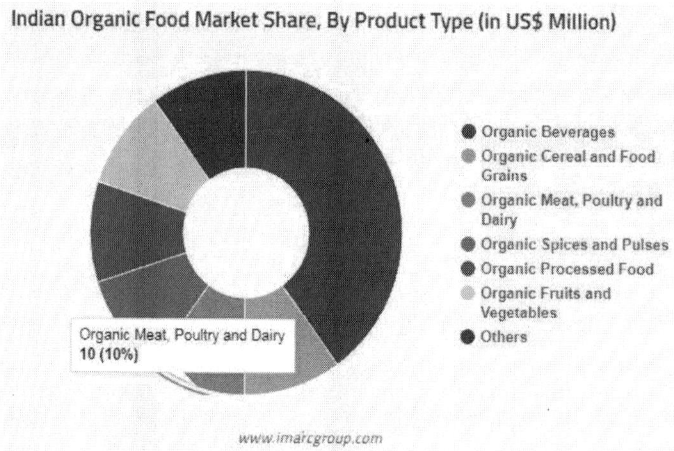

Organic Food Products & Consumers

The organic agricultural products including of livestock origin are gaining increasing popularity. The farmers can cash upon this growing interest in eco-friendly, animal welfare oriented, safe, nutritious and tastier meat products (as perceived by consumers of organic products). The eggs and meat obtained from such venture can be promoted as specialty item to restaurants; hotels and ethnic food jaunts fetching higher returns, better when local/*deshi* birdsare raised, which can better perform in free range system. Poultry can utilize the grazing lands/plantation areas (Rubber, coffee, coconut etc) by feeding on earth worms, small insects, green grass etc, while fertilizing the land with manure.

The free range poultry systems or pastured poultry is a sustainable agriculturetechnique that calls for the raising of laying chickens, broilers and turkeys on pasture, as opposed to indoor confinement. Humane treatment, the perceived health benefits of pastured poultry, in addition to superior texture and flavor, are causing an increase in demand for such products, which are believed to be having medicinal value, rich in antioxidants and least in chemical, medicinal or hormonal residues. Therefore, the growing interest in organic farming and meat & eggs drawn from free range systems might offer an attractive option in the form of market premiums for livestock farmers to venture into organic production.

Educating consumer and producer both is important to promote organic livestock production. Consumers need to be told that the safe milk and meat that they are looking for is the certified organic milk and meat, while farmers need to be made aware of this demand to be able for them to translate it into the new market opportunity. Also, there is a small but very concerned section of the society who does not consume livestock products owing to issues of animal cruelty, ill-treatment with them etc. The organic rearing of the farm animals sincerely addresses these issues and the certifiers approve that the due care has been taken in the process of production. These standards ensure that animals are kept free or never tied without specific purpose, allowed to express their physiological behaviour, fed with chemical free fodder, are not given hormonal injections and are reared in a completely stress free atmosphere. The information gap with respect to organic animal husbandry at the level of produces and consumers need to be bridged by suitable extension education interventions and encouraging the farmers, milk brands, cooperatives to enter this market on one side and consumers at the other end.

The Current Scenario

There are 52 certified organic dairy operators, 66 meat operators & 3 certified egg operators in India. The information on domestic sales of organic livestock products indicate the availability of certified organic milk and milk products in India (Table1). Also, India exported 2125.6 kg of certified organic *Ghee* (Clarifed butter) to UAE during 2019-20. Animals not only produce products for direct human consumption, but also help produce organic by-products like cattle urine & cow dung used to enhance soil fertility.

Table1: Production & sales of certified organic milk & milk products in India (2019-20).

S.No.	Item	Quantity MT(Metric Ton)
1.	Milk	16050
2.	Ghee (Clarified butter)	400
3.	Butter	9
4.	Milk Cream	390
5.	Skiimed Milk	320
6.	Skiimed milk powder	660

At ICAR-Indian Veterinary Research Institute as well as several other animal science research institutes and Veterinary Universities/colleges initiatives are underway to promote organic animal husbandry. For instance, the ICAR-National Research Centre on Meat got its organic sheep unit certified having the knowhow to handhold and guide the prospective farmers through all the processes involved in taking up organic sheep farming and certification.Out of total 32 accredited certification bodies (CBs) in India, 7 CBs are accredited for certification of livestock & poultry. It has taken initiatives to train certification bodies and evaluation committee to inspect & audit organic livestock operations. The author has been associated with all such capacity building programmes undertaken by APEDA to develop organic animal husbandry in India. Also, he has been training the Inspectors of certification bodies on certification process for organic livestock products. The start-ups, entrepreneurs including the farmers wishing to convert to organic animal husbandry need to be aware of the conversion, production & certification procedures for organic livestock production (Prakati 2020).

The Government of India is supporting several projects on organic agriculture that includes organic animal husbandry too. At the Agribusiness Incubation Cell (ABI) of ICAR- Indian Veterinary Research Institute, project proposals are invited for nurturing/incubating. The selected candidates are regularly mentored & financially supported to further develop the proposals including on organic production having market potential. They are trained on the topics like product development, branding, market assessment, launching in the market, winning consumers' confidence, product innovation, labeling, packaging, managemental aspects, record keeping etc. The trainees, wishing to start organic livestock and poultry production, are mentored through capacity building programmes. They are being introduced to the established certified organic farmers and export value-chains for awareness, knowledge and opportunities in the sector. The trainees are often very apprehensive of export markets for organic livestock products which have serious challenges mainly due to existence of infectious diseases in India like Foot & Mouth Disease (FMD) which restrict export to FMD free countries mostly in developed countries.

The capacity building initiatives on organic animal husbandry including mentoring of start-ups has been helping the farmers and entrepreneurs to get constructively engaged in enterprises related to organic livestock production. The startups are making organic food more accessible and affordable to the consumers, while creating new opportunities for farmers by motivating them to adopt organic livestock farming practices.Not only organic foods but the start-ups are engaged in producing value added products from animal by-products, which has attractive market in India and have possibilities of exports too. The initiatives have also been taken in India regarding certified organic sheep wool production. It would be better if pastoralist system prevailing in parts of country like barren mountainous regions/Islands/deserts/areas inhibited and managed by nomads are covered first under Participatory Guarantee System (PGS) and gradually switched to Third party certification considering the market potential of products from such areas and communities. The Sundarban in West Bengal is one good example, wherein, communities have been organized under Women Dairy Cooperative Societies and production of milk; milk products, honey etc have been certified and being marketed as 'certified organic'.

Landless Organic Animal Husbandry is Forbidden

Organic animal husbandry starts from the ground up. The basic requirement is more of a farm land than the cows or buffaloes. Organic farming including livestock production is basically a land based system, and landless animal husbandry system is forbidden in organic livestock farming. So, landless livestock farmers are not eligible for organic farming unless they go for land leasing. Farmers can raise suitable forage crops to feed their cattle and surplus can be marketed to needy farmers of that region. Forage crops should be grown without any chemical fertilizers and pesticides. Animal manure should be diverted to fields to maintain the fertility of the soil. There should be recycling of nutrients between plants and animals. In nutshell, the feed and fodder requirements have to be met on farm as far as possible. The landless farmers may find it difficult to meet this requirement of organic dairying, unless they have control on land for growing feed and fodder.

Selection of Breeds as a Prelude to Organic Farming

Farmer has to choose a breed that suits local conditions in terms of its disease resistance, maintenance cost and adaptability. There is no restriction on type of breeds, it could be exotic, crossbreeds or indigenous. If possible, pure breeds have to be maintained. A farmer can maintain an organic farm with local *desi* cattle whose genetic and production potential can be up-graded with bulls of good producing records, if necessary. Farmer can go for indigenous breeds which are proven for their genetic potential.

As per the organic standards, all animals should be born and raised on the organic holding. However, a beginner can procure calves from conventional farms, which are of 4 week old that received colostrum and full milk diet. In the same way, breeding stock to a maximum of yearly 10% can be brought in from conventional farms. Animal production record is important along with mothering ability, hardiness and thriftiness, resistance to disease and parasites, ability to forage etc., for which Indian native breeds are naturally endowed.

Farmers have to follow natural reproductive techniques. However, technique like artificial insemination is allowed, which is accepted to meet international standards of organic farming. Practices like embryo transfer technique, hormonal treatment, induced birth and genetically engineered breeds, which are high capital intensive, are not allowed in organic farming practices.

Housing as a Means of Providing Natural Habitation

Housing in organic farming should be according to the behavioral pattern of animals. Farmer should see that there is sufficient free movement with accessibility to fresh air and natural daylight besides protecting the animals from excessive sunlight and rain. Animal should have access to fresh water to meet its requirement. Herd animals shall not be kept individually and tethering is not allowed in organic farming. If tethering is to be done, it should allow the animal to move freely with sufficient space.

Space requirements for different category of cattle

S.No	Group of animals	Indoor Space m^2/ animal	Solid floor space (indoor) m^2/ animal	yard space (outdoor) m^2 / animal
1.	Breeding bulls	10.00	5.0	30.0
2.	Dairy cows	6.0	3.0	4.5
3.	Young stock < 100 kg	1.5	0.75	1.1
4.	101-200kg	2.5	1.25	1.9
5.	201-350kg	4.0	2.0	3.0
6.	350kg	5.0	2.5	3.7

Overcrowding shouldn't be done in order to avoid conflict behavior and associated health problems.

Feeding of Livestock in an Organic Farm

A farmer should feed an animal according to its physiological requirements. Diet should be according to animal's natural feeding behavior and digestive needs. Farmers should raise forage crops organically on their own, to feed the livestock. S/he should see to maximize production of feedstuffs on farm and the rate of success of organic farm depends on self-sufficiency in feed production. As a rule, 80% of feed should be from organic sources, however, at times of difficulties and emergencies, feed from conventional farm may be given with a dry matter content of 15% which has to be gradually reduced to 10% within 5 years.

When formulating rations, diet of animal should be balanced by adjusting the protein percentage to complement the forage levels. For example, when rations are based on high protein forage, care should be taken to ensure that energy levels are met by straw or hay to balance the excess protein. Growth regulators, artificial coloring agents, urea, medicated feeds, hormones, chemically extracted feeds, synthetic appetizers etc., are strictly prohibited in feeding the livestock of organic farm.

To supplement the feed of animals, plant based products, by-products of food industry like molasses; fodder preservatives like bacteria, fungal and enzymatic elements, vitamins, trace elements can be added as per requirement.

Raising of calf is more important, as it is the future organic milch animal. Calf be allowed to suckle according to its natural requirement and proper weaning be done unlike in conventional systems. In case of emergencies, calf may be given milk from non-organic farming systems or dairy substitutes so long as they contain neither antibiotics nor synthetic additives.

Preventive Management Plays a Major Role

Health care starts with selection of a breed, which has natural immunity against diseases and with good adaptability to local situation. Health care of livestock depends on the manner in which they are raised and the quality of feed offered, which result in maximum disease resistance. In organic livestock farming, preventive management plays major role and moreover, if any illness occurs, farmer should try to find out the cause, and change the managemental practices accordingly in order to prevent future outbreaks.

For treating the sick animals, farmer should give importance to natural medicines and methods including homeopathy, *ayurvedic* medicine and acupuncture. However, conventional medicines can be used, when no other alternative is available, as the well-being of the animal is the primary consideration in organic farming. But, if the animal is on allopathic treatment for two subsequent times, it looses the status of organic. Farmer can vaccinate his animals when diseases are known or expected to be a problem in the region that too with legally required vaccines only. Genetically engineered vaccines are prohibited. Instead of relying on medication, the farmer should strengthen the animal, so the immune system can do its job. So, farmer should be well aware that, health care in organic farming starts with selection of suitable breeds, raising the livestock according to its natural requirement; feeding good quality feed along with required grazing to strengthen the immune system of the animal and providing suitable housing to avoid related stress and associated health problems.

Record Maintenance - A must

Farmer has to maintain the records - right from the procurement of livestock, it's feeding, breeding, health care, production, till to the marketing of the product along with the type of labor involved (child labor is not allowed), method of processing, inputs to the farm and animal welfare measures taken which is a must for inspection purpose and certification of the farm and products as organic. Farmer should not be ignorant of this, in spite of his illiteracy and amazing memory, as it is a valuable tool for assessing the performance of one's herd or flock by the certifying agencies, which is mandatory for the milk to be labeled as 'organic'.

To bring a conventional farm to the organic status, the whole farm including milk & meat animals should be converted according to the standards set down (NPOP, 2015). The milk or meat can be sold as organic only after the farm has been under conversion for at least 12 months, provided the organic production standards have been met for the appropriate time. Once conformity with organic standards has been verified by a certification body, the product is accorded organic label which carries the name of the certification body and the standards with which it complies. To the informed consumer, this label functions as a guide and an assurance of purity. Certification bodies evaluate operations according to different organic standards and can be formally recognized by more than one authoritative body.

Marketing of Organic Products

Farm branded organic milk can serve as an effective way for a small producer to establish an identity and market niche and present possibilities for supplying to national and international markets. Development of other processed foods may itself create a demand for organic products such as milk powder or butter as ingredients in biscuits and confectionary. Structural organizations like co-operatives and farmers producer organizations can be effectively utilized for promotion of organic brands.

Conclusion

Organic animal husbandry research & developmental activities are largely concentrated in countries in EU and some other developed countries. Yet, developing countries like China, Mexico and Brazil are main exporting countries of eggs & Honey to EU. Bovine meat and non edible animal products are imported from Uruguay. Organic sheep and goat meat originate from New Zealand, while cheese is imported in EU from the USA (Willer et al 2021 & Chander et al 2011). This shows the potential for countries like India to export organic livestock products to EU and other developed countries. Certified Organic animal products are being supplied by several companies in India with growing demand. When the quality conscious consumers are looking for organic animal products, domestic sales and exports is picking up, it calls for efforts to promote organic animal husbandry.

The organic livestock and poultry standards have been notified in India for implementation since 1st June, 2015 (APEDA, 2015). It's the high time that attention is focused on organic animal husbandry including spreading the awareness on organic livestock and poultry standards through seminars, conferences and capacity building measures. It is important that stakeholders in India are acquainted with the concept, standards, practices, requirements and guidelines of organic livestock and poultry production, to improve their understanding of this emerging system of food production. The conventional poultry production with practices like rearing poultry in cages, feeding chemical laced feeds including antibiotics are considered not only against animal welfare but also seen as detrimental to human health and environment. Whereas, free range systems like backyard poultry production and extension sheep and goat husbandry are more welfare oriented and eco-friendly, so close to standards and guidelines set for organic livestock production. Organic agriculture is being seen as an alternative agricultural production system which has potential to make agriculture sustainable, protect environment and prevent or reduce the adverse impact of climate change. Organic agriculture including organic livestock and poultry production is an emerging system of food production, which is expanding rapidly around the world. Organic eggs have a decent market in many countries like USA UK, South Korea and China. Indian market for organic animal products is in budding stage, just emerging. With growing popularity, there is a lot of scope for organic production, marketing and consumption of milk, meat & eggs in India. The certified organic animal products offer potential opportunity for exports to many countries. This opportunity needs to be tapped.

References

Chander M., B. Subrahmanyeswari, Reena Mukherjee and S Kumar(2011): Organic livestock production: an emerging opportunity with new challenges to producers in tropical countries. Rev.Sci.Tech.Off. Int. Epiz, 30 (3), 969-983.

Chander Mahesh & B Subrahmanyeswari (2013): Organic Livestock Farming. Directorate of Knowledge Management in Agriculture, New Delhi, ICAR, 293p.

NPOP. 2024. National Programme for Organic Production (NPOP) Eigth Edition., Min. of Commerce and Industry, Department of Commerce, GoI New Delhi, 249p (https://npop.apeda.gov.in/sites/default/files/2024-10/NPOP_Eight_Edition_2024.pdf (Retrieved on 21st May, 2025)

Prakati (2020): 5 Organic Milk Startups in India. Prakati, July 2. https://www.prakati.in/5-organic-milk-startups-in-india/

PTI (2021): India's organic food products exports jump 51% to $1 bn in 2020-21. Business Today, June17. https://www.businesstoday.in/current/economy-politics/indias-organic-food-products-exports-jump-51-to-1-bn-in-2020-21/story/437718.html

Willer, Helga, Jan Trávníček and Bernhard Schlat t er (Eds.) (2025): The World of Organic Agricult ure.Statistics and Emerging Trends 2025. Research Institute of Organic Agriculture FiBL, Frick, and IFOAM – Organics International, Bonn.

3

Organic Goat Meat Production and Processing

Yogesh Gadekar, P Baswa Reddy and S.B. Barbuddhe

ICAR-National Meat Research Institute, Hyderabad, Telangana

Goats are the backbone of the Indian rural economy as it helps in sustaining the livelihood of rural poor in difficult terrains. The value output from the sheep and goat meat sector has been worth Rs123177 crores during 2020-2021 (Central Statistical Organisation, GoI). India has diverse small ruminant genetic resources with 44 sheep and 37 goat breeds registered with the ICAR National Bureau of Animal Genetic Resources, Karnal. The goat population has colossally increased by 215% (47.2 vs 148.9 million) from 1951 to 2019. Of late, the last two censuses revealed that the goat population in the country increased by 10.1% (135.17 to 148.88 million). The goats are 27.8% of the total livestock population in the country. Their contribution to total meat production is 13.63%. The goat and sheep contributed 1467 million kg of meat in 2021-22 (BAHS, 2022). Goat meat is increasing and is mostly preferred in North and Western India. Meat consumption in India is showing an upward trend but still, there is a lot of scope for improvement in per capita availability. The global Covid-19 pandemic altered the food preferences of the consumer with more demand for safe foods produced under the natural system. The organic food production system may be aptly suited and has potential to meet out demands of consumers. This change in the consumer attitude is gradually increasing the scope and opening more avenues for organic food production and marketing. Food safety legislation in different countries is also working towards improving the safety standards of food and, at the same time, consumers are increasingly willing to pay for quality foods as their disposable incomes rise.

Organic Food Production

Organic production has seen a phenomenal growth trajectory during the past two decades. India with 2.30 million organic producers has the most number of organic farmers in the world. Total organic cultivation area, 27, 59,660 total farmers (11, 60,650 PGS and 15, 99,010 India Organic), 1703 total processors, and 745 traders. A major relative increase in organic agricultural land was noted in the recent past throughout the country (https://ncof.dacnet.nic.in/StatusOrganicFarming). The number of food categories sold as organic is growing rapidly in India. Starting with organic tea and spices, it's grown to organic flour, breakfast cereals, fruits, vegetables, and many more. Of late, the consumer demand for organically produced livestock products like milk, eggs, and meat is also on the rise.

In India, the domestic organic food products market is growing at around 20% CAGR in recent years. During 2020-21 in India, there were around 16 lakh organic producers under the NPOP production system producing 34.9 lakh tons of organic products in 43.3 lakh hectares of land including 16.8 lakh hectares under wild harvest. During this period, 8.88 lakh tons of organic products worth Rs.7078 crores were exported from India. Under Participatory Guaranty System (PGS) in India, as of September 2021, there are about 42 thousand organic farmer groups comprising around 12 lakh farmers producing organic products on 75 lakh hectares of land. Madhya Pradesh, Maharashtra, Karnataka, Rajasthan, and Uttar Pradesh are the major organic production states in the country and the major commodities produced are oil seeds, fibre, sugar, cereals, millets, spices, and condiments. USA, EU, Canada, and Australia are major export destinations of Indian organic products, and the major organic products exported from India are processed foods, oil seeds, cereals, millets, spices, and tea.Though the organic crop production and certification system are reasonably well established in India, the organic livestock and poultry sector is in its infancy. Organizations such as APEDA, FSSAI and BIS along with research establishments like ICAR- National Meat Research Institute, Hyderabad are now putting serious efforts to establish the protocols and promote organic livestock production and certification in India. As a result, in the last few years, livestock farmers are gradually getting encouraged to take up organic production, and around 3000 farmers mostly from Uttar Pradesh, Madhya Pradesh, and Himachal Pradesh have taken up organic dairy, sheep, and poultry farming. Organic milk and ghee from India are now being exported to different countries.

Organic Meat Production

Organic livestock production and marketing of organic livestock products like milk, meat, and eggs have witnessed an upward trend in the growth rate worldwide in the last decade. The global organic meat products market is expected to grow from USD 15 billion in 2020 to USD 20 billion in 2025 at a CAGR of around 7%. In India, the organic meat sector is yet to take off. A few organic sheep, poultry, and pig units have recently been established and the certified organic meat from these units is likely to enter the markets in the next couple of years. The organic animal production system is emerging as an effective alternative to address all these issues. Owing to this, in India, there are bright prospects for tapping this opportunity to develop it into a business model in the Animal Husbandry sector.

Goat meat which is a highly sought-after meat in India, especially in the northern states, has the niche scope to cater to health-conscious consumers. However, enlightenment of the goat farmers about the scope of organic farming and the promotion of certified organic meat are the initial hurdles to overcome before this sector takes off in the country. ICAR- National Meat Research Institute, Hyderabad has taken initiative in this regard and established the first NPOP-certified organic sheep unit in the country to serve as a model unit for enthusiastic entrepreneurs to take up activities in the certified organic sheep and goat meat sector.

Organic Livestock Production Standards

The broad guidelines for organic livestock production under the National Programme for Organic Production (NPOP) of India are as under:

a) *Organic management plan:* Before starting organic livestock farming, the producer has to make a detailed organic management plan and present it to the certifying agency for approval.

b) *Breed /Strain selection:* Local breeds/strains which can easily be acclimatized to local climatic conditions shall be preferred over the exotic breeds

c) *Source / Origin:* Initial stock should be sourced from organically certified units. If the animals are introduced from non-organic units, they should undergo a mandatory conversion period as specified for each category of livestock.

d) *Housing and management:* Livestock shall be maintained under natural conditions as far as possible. This shall include utilizing natural breeding methods, housing, and management conditions tominimize stress, a health management system to prevent diseases. Minimum shaded as well as open areas as specified for each category of livestock shall be followed.

e) *Conversion period:* Animals brought from non-organic sources shall undergo a conversion period as specified for each category of livestock and poultry. During the conversion period, the animals should be maintained under organic conditions. After completion of the conversion period, the animals can be sold as organic. In case of small ruminants conversion period is 6 months for meat and milk purpose.

f) *Feeding:* Livestock shall be provided with organically produced feed during the entire rearing period. The agricultural land committed for the cultivation of feed/fodder crops intended to be used as feed for livestock shall be organic. The overall feeding practices shall satisfy the daily nutrient requirements of the concerned animals. Feed additives and supplements used for feeding shall be from natural sources and as permitted under organic livestock guidelines.

g) *Healthcare:* Organic livestock, in general, should follow the basic principles of preventive health and productivity management wherein the focus would be on preventing diseases, detecting underlying fertility and production problems, and its correction primarily on correcting management, nutrition, and sanitation. Antibiotics and other allopathic drugs are not permitted. For purpose of treatment and prevention of diseases and under-performances, herbal/ phytotherapeutic (excluding antibiotics), homeopathic or ayurvedic products shall be preferred to allopathic veterinary drugs or antibiotics, provided that their therapeutic effect is effective for the species of animal and the condition for which the treatment is intended.Antibiotics and other allopathic drugs can be used when other modes of cure are not effective to save the life of the animal and in such cases, withdrawal periods as prescribed for each drug should be strictly followed. Hormonal treatment and use of growth promotors shall not be permitted. All vaccinations required by law of the land shall be permitted.

h) *Breeding and Management:* The preference for reproduction shall be through natural methods, although artificial insemination may be used. Embryo transfer techniques and the use of hormonal reproductive treatment shall not be used unless prescribed for therapeutic purposes directed towards correcting the physiological problem. The breeding techniques employing genetic engineering shall not be used.

i) *Manure and urine management:* Manure and urine excreta collection and management practices in the organic livestock & poultry farm are critical components. The collection, handling, and disposal of the dung andurine from the shed, paddock, open run, or grazing areas shall be implemented in a manner that minimizes soil and water degradation, does not significantly contribute to contamination of water, optimizes recycling of nutrients and does not include burning or any practice inconsistent with organic practices.

j) *Transport:* During transport, the producer shall prevent stress, injury, hunger, thirst, malnutrition, fear, distress, physical & thermal discomfort, pain, and diseaseduring the transport and shall observe all the conditions set in law of the land for animal transportation. Animals must be fit for the intended journey. All necessary arrangements shall be made in advance to minimize the length of the journey and meet the animal's needs during the journey. Means of transport, as well as the loading and unloading facilities, must be designed, constructed, maintained, and operated to avoid injury and suffering and ensure the safety of the animals.

k) *Slaughter:* The slaughter of livestock and poultry shall be undertaken in a manner, which minimizes stress and suffering, and shall be following the territorial/ national rules framed for the purpose. The minimum age of slaughter for each species of livestock should be followed as prescribed for the respective species.

Organic Livestock Certification

Production of crops or livestock organically without validation or auditing has limited reach to the consumers. Certification of organic products and processes serves this purpose and improves consumer confidence and thereby widening the market for organic produce. Farmers interested in organic farming need to assess the pros and cons of each system of certification and choose the one which fulfills their requirements.

The different avenues of organic certification in India are

1. National Programme for Organic Production (NPOP)

The National Programme for Organic Production (NPOP) certification system of India involves a third-party inspection to ascertain the compliance of the organic production system. The certification is supervised by the APEDA at the national level. APEDA authorizes the eligible certification agencies through a process of accreditation and these certification bodies can take up the certification at the farm/producer/processor/grower group level. The produce certified under NPOP is entitled to carry the 'India Organic' logo along with the 'Jaivik Bharat' logo as specified by FSSAI and can be sold within India and also can be exported to other countries as organic product after complying with the requirements of the importer.

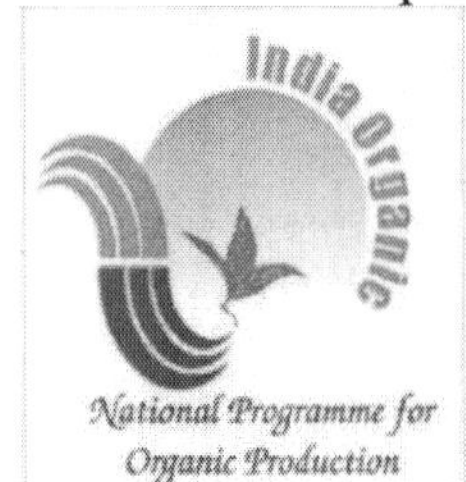

2. Participatory Guarantee System (PGS)

Participatory Guarantee System (PGS) is a quality assurance initiative that is locally relevant, emphasizes the participation of stakeholders, including producers and consumers, and operates outside the frame of third-party certification. This certification is based on the active participation of stakeholders and is built on a foundation of trust, social networks, and knowledge exchange. It is for farmers or communities that can organize and perform as a group within the village or in close-by villages with continuous territory. PGS ensures traceability only up to the end till it is in the custody of the group. Once the product leaves the custody of the PGS group there is no control of PGS over its integrity. The produce certified under PGS can use the logo of 'PGS-Green' (for farm/ produce under conversion) or 'PGS- Organic' (for farm/ produce completely concerted to Organic) along with the Jaivik Bharat logo as specified by FSSAI and can be sold within India as an organic product.

PGS-INDIA
GREEN
Logo Used while marketing on the products produced from the field under conversion
PGS-INDIA
ORGANIC
Logo Used while marketing on the products produced from fields of completely converted into organic

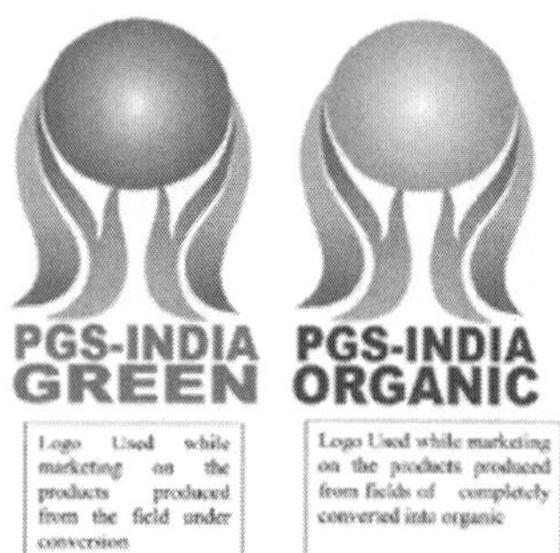

Certified organic fodder production or certification of grazing land is in similar lines to the certification of crops which is fairly established in India. Organic certification of livestock products (value-added products of meat, milk, etc.,) is considered in a similar category as that of certification of processed foods and other value-added food products which requires organic processing certification.The process of becoming organically certified can be expensive, but it is an essential step for farmers and manufacturers wanting to meet the growing demand for certified organic food among quality-conscious consumers which fetches a premium price for their produce.

Promotion of Organic Production by the Government

The Government of India has introduced multiple schemes and incentives to encourage the adoption of organic farming by farmers. The most prominent schemes of the government for the promotion of organic farming in India areParamparagatKrishiVikasYojana (PKVY), Mission Organic Value Chain Development in NE Region (MOVCDNER) National Project on Organic Farming (NPOF), Rashtriya KrishiVikasYojana (RKVY), Mission for Integrated Development of Horticulture (MIDH), ICAR-Network Project on Organic farming, NamamiGange Project, etc. ParamparagatKrishiVikasYojana (PKVY) is an elaborated component of Soil Health Management (SHM) of the major project National Mission of Sustainable Agriculture (NMSA).

Challenges

a) *Awareness:* Lack of awareness among the farmers about the guidelines of organic livestock & poultry farming and the processes available for their certification is the main hurdle hindering the development of this sector in the country.

b) *Certification:* Very few organic certifying agencies in India have accreditation for livestock certification. In the case of organic crop certification under PGS, in many states, the machinery of state agricultural departments is involved in organic certification but the same is lacking in the case of livestock certification.

c) *Labour:* Currently, organic food production is assumed to be more labour intensive since under this system the farmers are advised to be more animal welfare friendly and adopt traditional health care systems which involve relatively higher labour when compared to allopathic health care.

d) *Documentation:* Documentation of all the processes and activities in organic production and marketing of the produce under the NPOP system is a cumbersome process for an ordinary farmer

e) *Productivity:* Initially, the productivity of organic livestock farms is likely to be lower than thatof traditional commercial farms till the organic livestock management, nutrition, health care, and reproduction practices are fine-tuned for higher production yields.

f) *Costs:* Organic certification is expensive and organic feed for animals can cost twice that of normal feed. Organic farms tend to be smaller than conventional farms, which means fixed costs and overhead must be distributed across smaller produce volumes without government subsidies.

g) *Market:* Organised market for organic livestock products is yet to evolve in the country. Since there is no stringent enforcement mechanism, certified organic produce has to face competition from non-certified and dubious produce sold in the market.

However, as the markets for organic products get matured and certified organic livestock products gain consumer confidence, these products fetch premium prices which can nullify the higher costs involved in production and certification.

Issues in Organic Livestock Production and Certification

- Double certification (for animals and fodder)
- Weak PGS mechanism for organic livestock certification
- Organic Feed availability and cost
- Healthcare expertise through Ayurvedic and Homeopathic medication
- Tagging of Animals
- Slaughter and processing facilities
- False Organic claims
- Awareness creation
- Cost of certification for small holders

Since organic livestock rearing and organic livestock product preparation are yet to leap in India, there are vast opportunities in all stages of the organic value chain right from production through certification, value addition, and marketing till consumption. All the products and services in the organic food value chain are likely to fetch a premium price in the market as they are targeted at niche consumers who are quality conscious and would be willing to pay a premium price for quality products. The demand for organic chevon would certainly rise with increasing awareness and purchasing power of the consumers. Further, this sector has huge potential for employment generation and increasing farmer's income.

4

Traditional Designer Goat Milk and Meat Products: Processing and Quality Assurance

Manish Kumar Chatli and Tarun Pal Singh

ICAR-Central Institute for Research on Goats, Makhdoom P.O. Farah-281122

Mathura, Uttar Pradesh Livestock plays a crucial role in agriculture and rural economies, affecting livelihoods, food security, public health, and economic development. The Gross Value Added (GVA)of livestock sector is about Rs. 11,14,249 crore at current prices during FY 2020-21 which is about 30.87%of Agricultural and Allied Sector GVA and 6.17%of Total GVA. At constant prices (2011-12), the GVA of livestock sector is about Rs. 6,17,117crore during FY2020-21with a positive growth of 6.13% over previous financial year (DAHD, 2022).Livestock contributed 16% to the income of small farm households that indicates importance of livestock sector as a whole. Despite the presence of limited land and water resources, India has the world's largest livestock population accounting for over 35.94% of cattle, 20.45% of buffalo, 26.40% of goats and 12.17% of sheep of the world's population. The goat population in the country was 148.88 million in 2019, increased by 10.1% over previous census BAHS, 2012 (DAHD, 2019).In India the goat sector contributes 8.4 percent to the Indian livestock GDP that is 1,16,400 crores through meat Rs64,000 crores, through milk 22000 crores, through skin Rs3345 crores, through manure Rs2535 crores, and others Rs4360 crores. India rank first in goat population and possessregistered37 goat breedsin different agro-climatic zones.Goats (*Capra hircus*) are one of the oldest domesticated species and it provides meat (Chevon), milk, *yoghurt*, cheese and other by-products such as hair and skin. Goats rearing provide much needed livelihood support to the landless and weaker sections and also hold considerable potential for commercializationas well as provide job opportunities in rural India. The goatsrequire lower feed and capital requirements thanlarge ruminants, so this is best suited for small and medium producers.It produces 2.93% milk and

13.67% meat of total meat production across the country. The goat population in the country is expected to reach to 216 million in 2050 with milk and skin production to 9.8 and 1.44 million tonnes, respectively. Goats are primarily used for meat production, both for domestic consumption and for export purposes.The nutritive value of goat meat as well as other food items like milk is becoming increasingly important in the health management of people. Since ancient times goat milk has traditionally been known for its medicinal properties and has recently gained importance in human health due to its proximity to human milk for easy digestibility and it's all round health promoting traits. There are over a billion people affected by the low protein food however goats can provide nutritional security to the poor farmers, rural women and children. Moreover, the increasing demand for goat milk and meat products could be fulfilled by increasing the animal numbers, increasing per animal productivity by providing optimum feeding, better management practices and proper health care management using latest innovative technologies pertaining to goats.

Goat Meat

In India, small ruminant meat is the most popular and highest-priced meat, and that is the biggest strength of this sector.In India, meat production has considerably increased over the last few decades.Although, with vegetarian diets supported by strong cultural and religious traditions, India has the lowest level of meat consumption in the world.The per capita meat consumption in India is estimated at 5.5 kg per year, which is about 50% of that recommended by the Indian Council of Medical Research. In 2022-23, the country produced 9.30 million tonnes of total meat, and goats contributing 1.27MT accounts for 13.67% (DAHD, 2021, 2022).Despite a large small ruminant population their productivity is low accounting dressing weight of only 10-12 kg as against 17 kg of worlds average.The slaughter rate was recorded as 74.82 % (111.32/148.4 million heads) in case of goats(BAHS, 2022). The carcass yield of small ruminants in India is relatively low as compared to the world average due to lack of proper feeding and low genetic merit as well as non-descript in nature. The productivity of indigenous breeds is lower than the exotic breeds. The leader country in goat meat production in the world is China.The percentage share of chevon production in different states is as follows: West Bengal > U.P. > Maharashtra > Bihar > Rajasthan > Odisha >Telengana> T.N. > Andhra Pradesh. During the year 2021-22 India was the largest exporter of sheep & goat meat to the world. The country has exported 8,695.97 metric tonnes of sheep & goat meat to the world for the worth of Rs. 447.58 Crores (APEDA, 2022). During 2021-22, the percent share of top five destination for sheep and goat meatwere United Arab Emirates (75.34%), Qatar (10.05%), Kuwait

(6.67%), Maldives (2.74%), and Oman (1.69%)(APEDA, 2022).Still, there is huge demand of Indian chilled fresh meat in South Asia and Gulf region due to natural goat rearing practices followed in India, which make it nearly organic.

Table 1: Export of Indian sheep/goat meat to different countries (APEDA, 2022)

S.No.	Countries	2020-21		2021-22		2021-22 % share
		Qty (MT)	Value (Rs. Lacs)	Qty (MT)	Value (Rs. Lacs)	
1.	UAE	5,226.62	24,799.52	6,401.40	33,720.29	75.34
2.	Qatar	717.95	3,505.20	825.69	4,498.67	10.05
3.	Kuwait	385.35	1,829.29	573.84	2,986.35	6.67
4.	Maldives	180.35	557.90	385.48	1,228.15	2.74
5.	Oman	230.61	886.47	180.89	885.22	1.98
6.	Saudi Arab	206.21	960.07	194.64	757.58	1.69
7.	Baharain	92.47	418.28	118.79	617.82	1.38
8.	Seychelles	8.22	32.37	13.59	56.80	0.13
9.	Nepal	1.71	3.59	0.00	0.00	0.00
10.	Others	1.06	3.68	1.65	6.81	0.02
	Total	**7,050.55**	**32,996.37**	**8,695.97**	**44,757.69**	**100**

Processing and Value Addition of Goat Meat

The meat production has registered a healthy growth. However, there is very little processing. Hardly 1% of the total meat produced in the country is used for processing and remaining meat is sold in fresh or frozen form. Very little of the meat consumed in India is pre-processed. An estimate of the Ministry of Food Processing Industries (MOFPI) suggests that the level of processing of meat in India is just about 6%, which includes pork and beef.Processing of meat serves primarily to add value to meat, give consumers variety and convenience, create employment, utilize low-value meat cuts and by-products from slaughterhouses more effectively, extend shelf life, incorporate non-meat ingredients, increase marketing and distribution, gain more profits, and expand export opportunities.A trail of Indian research has been traced around the processing of products and adding value to them.Emulsion technology supports the production of quality meat products through the use of tough meat and meat by-products from spent animals. Emulsion meatproducts like *nuggets, balls, sausages, kofta* and *patties*etc. and non-emulsion based traditional products such as *kebabs, pickle, samosa, cutlets and tikka* etc. can be prepared on a cottage scale using simple appliances.Better research understandings with the role in safety needs to be establishedbefore entering in to the international market. There is a need of designing products that haveparticular functional value to address a particular disease or symptom. It has been expected that in the functional aspect maystrengthen meat processing sector rapidly. ICAR-Central Institute for Research on Goats is continuously striving for the development of processing technology of goat meat products. The Institute has developed number of technologies for goat meat products, including emulsion-based products, ground product, shelf-stable product and functional meat products

In order to produce goat meat products sustainably, the private sector and government must commit to responsible stewardship of natural resources. Marketability of value added products and their research needs are to be prioritised for the support thesustainability of the new players.Producers are also looking for the international market. Though the market gap in terms of difference in rates are stillreported to be very narrow especially for the international market scenario.

Goat Milk

India occupies the first position in goat milk production (3.24% of totalmilk) largest milk contributing species after cow and buffaloes (DAHD 2019). The milk production from goats hasincreased from 3.26 million tonnes in 2000-01 to 6.09 million tonnes in 2018–19. The top

five goat milk production states are Rajasthan, Uttar Pradesh, Madhya Pradesh, Gujarat andMaharashtra accounting for 79.5% of total goat milk production. The goat milk sector in India has not received attention and is marketed largely through theinformal channel. The estimated global dairy goat population was 218 million in the year2017. Generally, goat breeds such as Beetal, Jamunapari, Jakhrana, Sirohi, Barbari, Jhalawadi and Surti found in the north and central part of India have higher milk yield (Chawla et al., 2009). The goat milk production in 2022 as 6.3 million metric tonnes and constituted 2.93 % of total milk production. The production of goat milk is expected to rise in the years ahead and it is projected that the goat milk production in the country by 2050 will be more than 10 million tonnes (Anon, 2013).

Table 2: Top goat milk-producing countries in the world (FAO, 2020)

Country	Goat milk (1000 Mt)	Percent of total milk
India	6098.37	3.24
Sudan	1151.00	25.07
Bangladesh	1122.65	55.61
Pakistan	915.00	1.99
France	652.33	2.46
Turkey	561.83	2.54
Mali	526.13	24.80
Spain	461.38	5.68
Greece	397.79	20.95
Somalia	374.87	17.43

Therapeutic Potential of Goat Milk

Goat milk was recognised in the ancient time, and it had a wide range of applications besides being used as a healthy food. However, in the era of industrial revolution consumer shifted their attention towards cow due to the production of bulk quantity of milk, which was regarded as convenient for the collection, transportation and processing. Goat milk has started receiving significant attention among researchers as well as consumers due to its inherent compositional and medicinal edge over other milk.The significance of goat milk in infant diet is very much appreciated on account of its easy digestibility and less allergic than cow milk. In goat milk the absence of agglutinin combined with the presence of higher short and medium-chain fatty acids prevents the fat globules clustering and making it easier to digest. Goat milk is also known to form a finer curd than cow milk following acidification, which mimics the conditions in the stomach, suggesting its rapid digestibility (Park, 2007). The low levels of αs_1-casein in goat milk and a higher proportion of β-casein suggest that the goat milk casein profile is much closer to human milk than cow milk (Clark and Sherbon, 2000). The relative absence of αs1-casein contributes to enhance the digestion of β-lactoglobulin (Bevilacqua et al., 2001).Medium chain triglycerides (MCT) and proteins occur more in goat milk, and have been recognized as unique lipids and proteins with unique health benefits. Due to the difference in goat milk's fat content, goat milk products have a softer texture, better digestibility for humans, and efficient lipid metabolism.As goat milk contains a high content of MCT, it seems likely that this is metabolized much more quickly to generate energy, since MCT is a highly available energy substrate. Compared to cow milk proteins, goat milk proteins are easier to digest. Goat milk typically contains 4-5 times higher oligosaccharides than cow milk and have important roles as prebiotics, which stimulate growth of the probiotic bacteria in the gastrointestinal tract. Goat milk has higher calcium, phosphorus, potassium, magnesium, and chlorine, and lower sodium and sulphur contents than cow milk.

Table 3: Healthier component of goat milk and their functions

S.N.	Component	Description	Functions
1.	Fat	Goat milk fat globules are smaller in size in comparison to cow milk. ~80% of fat globules are <5 µm in goat milk and ~60% in cow milk. A higher proportion of medium-chain triglycerides (36%), monounsaturated fatty acids (MUFA) and polyunsaturated fatty acids (PUFA), minor branched-chain fatty acids and lower content of trans-C18:1 fatty acid.	Forms soft textured curd with higher digestibility. Medium-chain triglycerides (MCT) have become established medical treatments for an array of clinical disorders. Higher MCT, MUFA and PUFA, and lower trans fatty acids are beneficial in the maintenance of cardiovascular health.
2.	Nucleotides	Goat milk has a complex array of nucleotides. Infant formula made from goat milk has same level of nucleotides as human milk (Prosser et al., 2008).	Immune maturation of milk-fed offspring, mediation of energy metabolism, signal transduction and general regulation of cell growth, lipoprotein metabolism, enhancement of high-density lipoprotein (HDL) plasma concentration, synthesis of apolipoprotein (Apo) A1 and Apo A1 V in pre-term infants, and upregulation of long-chain polyunsaturated fatty acid synthesis in human neonates (Schaller et al., 2007).
3.	Taurine	The amount of taurine in goat milk is 20-40 folds higher than cow milk (Silanikove et al., 2010).	Involved in bile salt formation, osmoregulation, antioxidation, calcium transport and functioning of the central nervous system (Silanikove et al., 2010). Regulate blood pressure and alleviate other cardiovascular ailments (Militante and Lombardini, 2002).
4.	Polyamines	Rich in goat colostrum and milk compared to milk of other mammals (Ploszaj et al., 1997).	Optimise growth, gastrointestinal tract (GIT) cell function, maturation of GIT enzymes (Silanikove et al., 2010) and reduce the incidence of food allergy in infants (Dandrifosse et al., 2000).

S.N.	Component	Description	Functions
5.	Oligosaccharides	Oligosaccharides in goat milk are 4-5 times higher than cow milk and 10 times higher than sheep milk.	Antiadhesive, antimicrobial, immune modulators, intestinal epithelial cell response modulation, nutrient for neonatal brain development and growth of desired gut microflora (Lima et al., 2018).

Processing and Value Addition of Goat Milk

Goat milk in India is mostly consumed either in the households or sold to the local market after mixing with the cow or buffalo milk (Agnihotri and Pal, 1996). It is really hard to find any goat milk products in Indian markets. Several goat milk products like paneer, khoa, shrikhand, cheeses, etc., have been developed in India however, barely adopted by the consumers and find a place in the market or poorly marketed. Lack of detailed studies on the preference of consumers' for goat milk products could be one of the reasons. To boost the Indian dairy goat farming there is a need to follow the success of Mediterranean countries in production and processing of goat milk and its value addition. In comparison to cow and buffalo milk, there are limited reports on goat milk products (Jandal 1996; Haenlein, 2004) possibly due to scattered research. Still, some works on dairy goat products have been reported (Park, 2005; Park and Guo, 2006a, b). According to Pandya and Ghodke (2007), availability of small volume of goat milk for commercial production is one of reasons for lower interest in goat milk products. Different goat milk products like dry whole milk, dried granulated milk, condensed goat milk, fruit *yoghurt*, cheeses, butter and butter oil, cultured goat cream butter, ice cream, whey protein concentrate, evaporated milk, traditional Indian products and Turkish butter have been reported (Park and Guo, 2006a, b; Pandya and Ghodke, 2007).

Quality Assurance

Goat products(milk, meat and their products)are generally regarded as high risk commodity in respect of pathogen contents, natural toxins and other possible contaminants and adulterants. These products have been major global causes of foodborne disease in humans and are also prone to microbiological growth and spoilage. Consequently, monitoring the safety and quality of these products remains a primary worldwide concern. Recognizing this, the World Health Organization (WHO) developed its Global Strategy for Food Safety (Adak et al., 2005). Indian milk and meat market are disruptive and unorganised. Majority of the products are sold fresh and without packaging. Therefore, the quality assurance becomes imperative for the safety of the consumer.

CIRG has developed SOPs for Clean Goat Milk and Meat Production. These guidelines are disseminated through various training programs, and literature to the stake holders. FSSAI has issued the standards for fresh and processed meat products, which should be followed by the processors.

Conclusions

The low productivity or carcass yield can be addressed by selection of goat breeds for meat product, cross breeding with superior germplasm, organized goat farming for meat production and improve slaughter infrastructure as well as personnel training. Attempts should be made to upgrade other Indian goat breeds to increase their milk yield by well-known improver breeds. Improvement in goat milk production will not only fulfil domestic protein requirement of rural peoples but also create avenue for employment and income. ICAR-CIRG has endeavoured in this regard and come out with number of commercially viable goat meat and milk product. Also, the therapeutic potential of goat milk is becoming recognized because of the medicinal values for treating many human diseases. Hopefully such technologies will to the industry and more goat meat products will reach out to the market. The concerted efforts will be made at all levels for the development of dairy goat sector and one day India would be one of the major global players in the field of goat milk and milk products.

5

Role of Livestock in Food Security in India: With Special Reference to Goat Farming

Maya Kant Awasthi

Centre for Food and Agribusiness Management, Indian Institute of Management Lucknow, Uttar Pradesh

Indian farming community is dominated by the marginal and small farmers who account for nearly 86 percent of farm holdings in India. As these farmers have small land holdings of less than 2 hectare, their income from farming is meagre and not sufficient to meet family expenses (Lalji et al., 2019). As a result, these farmers often follow family income augmentation strategy either by taking land on lease, working as wage earner or livestock rearing. Among all these family income augmentation activities, livestock rearing is the most frequently adopted strategy they undertake to augment their family income. It is observed that in India in general, farmers follow livestock integrated farming system (Paramesh et al, 2022). Popularity of livestock activity to augment farm family income of poor farmers is due to synergy of livestock rearing with the farming. Agriculture waste in the form of green and dry fodder contribute important inputs in livestock rearing. Whereas, farm animals are important source of farm energy needed for cultivation. Livestock waste helps in maintaining soil fertility and protein supply to farm families. Animal rearing also help in managing cash flow for farm family as it generates cash from the sale of milk and other animal products on the daily basis. Sale of live animals help in meeting contingency expenses of farm family. Thus, it solves peculiar problem of farm family cash paradox where farmer gets income through sales of agriculture harvest only during harvest season which happens only two / three times in a year but he needs cash on daily basis to meet his other health, educational, social etc. family needs.

It is observed that livestock rearing is becoming increasingly difficult for poor farmers due to rising cost of inputs required for livestock rearing. These farmers therefore often shift from the cattle rearing to goat rearing as goats can survive in harsh environment and will need little input and care but have high income generation potential (Lalljee et al., 2019).

Role of Livestock in Food Security

In the year, 2008 FAO identified availability of food products, accessibility, food quality and food safety as four critical dimensions of the food security. Achieving these food security dimensions are critical for realising food security. Latter sustainability was also included as the long-term time fifth dimension of food security. Sustainability of production is critical for maintaining capabilities of future generations and their food security (Berry et al., 2015). Therefore, the key requirements for achieving food security for the poor is that whenever he need, required food should not only be available to him but he should also have physical and economic access to healthy good quality food throughout the year produced by a sustainable production system. Goat farming can help him in achieving this through goat rearing induced improved and sustainable cash flow which results in improved purchasing power.

Managing the impact of goat rearing on all economic, social, ecological and governance subsystems of local eco system is also not very difficult to manage and therefore this activity of income augmentation is compatible with the sustainable development, doubling farmers income and food security etc. policy goals of Government.

Marketing Based Optimisation of Goat Value Chain for Food Security

Traditionally in food chain, value is created through either adding place value, time value or through changes in the form of the product. Significant research has been conducted on these three forms of value addition or value optimization through these methods. However, most of the time we ignore value creation potential of marketing activity. In marketing, value is created through optimizing value perception of the product through effective marketing communication. Value perception of the product can be also achieved by incorporating non tangible product attributes like organic nature of product, convenience, traceability, quality and safety assurance in the product design.

Value chain management in international trade is another key area which has high potential due to high price differential in domestic and international products. However, for this we must manage following impediments of international value chain.

- Non-tariff barriers
- Food safety standard
- HACCP, Codex, GAP, ISO
- Traceability
- Value perception

After signing of Agreement on Agriculture (AoA) in World Trade Organisation (WTO) in the year 1995, discriminating agriculture producers located outside the country to protect domestic producers has become difficult. As opening the domestic market for outside producers and providing them non-discriminatory treatment has become mandatory for every country. In such a situation, most of the developed countries have started using arbitrary quality standards or Phyto sanitary conditions to stop exporter from exporting their products and protecting their domestic players. WTO has provided mechanism to appeal for such trade distortion practices. But appeals for such cases takes years before it is settled and thus provided few years protection to domestic producer from the competition. These non-tariff barriers are biggest impediments in realising full potential of international value chain of livestock products such as goat and sheep.

Impact of Goat Value Chain on Food Security

Integration of livestock with farming specially with small ruminant such as goat has positive impact on production and productivity, resource use efficiency and sustainability. It has positive impact on food availability, physical and economic access to food and quality and safety of food available and sustainability of food production system at the farm family level. Impact path of livestock rearing on food security has been explained in figure 1.

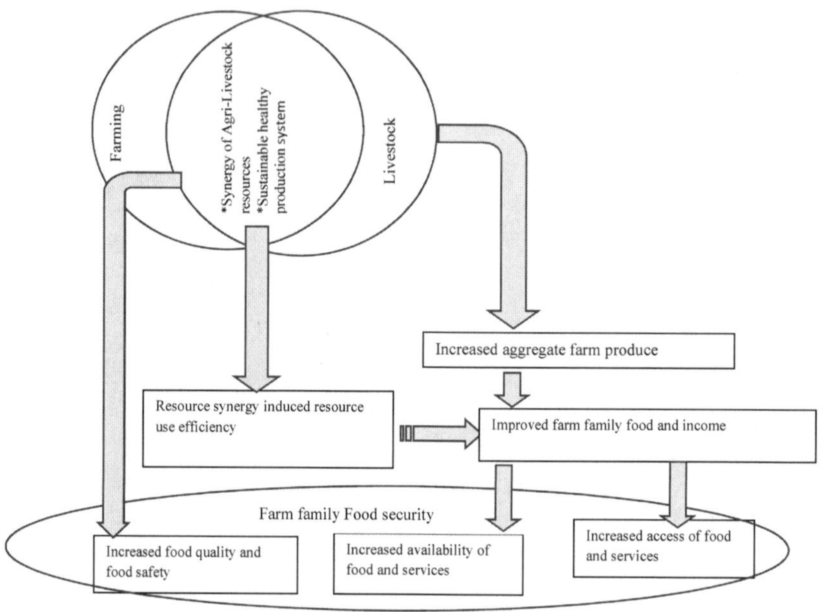

Fig. 1: Impact of integrating Livestock enterprise with agriculture on food security

References

Berry, E.M., Dernini, S., Burlingame, B., Meybeck, A., Conforti, P., 2015. Food security and sustainability: can one exist without the other? Public Health Nutr. 18, 2293–2302.

FAO, 2008. Food Security Information for Action: Practical Guides. EC - FAO Food Security Programme, Rome. FAO, 2009.

Lalljee, S. V., Soundararajan, C., Singh, Y. D., & Sargison, N. D. (2019). The potential of small ruminant farming as a means of poverty alleviation in rural southern India. *Tropical animal health and production*, *51*, 303-311.

Paramesh, V., Ravisankar, N., Behera, U., Arunachalam, V., Kumar, P., Solomon Rajkumar, R., ... & Rajkumar, S. (2022). Integrated farming system approaches to achieve food and nutritional security for enhancing profitability, employment, and climate resilience in India. *Food and Energy Security*, *11*(2), e321.

6

Traditional Veterinary Medicine and Technologies for Natural Animal Farming

Ashok Kumar, Anu Rahal, Ravindra Kumar, Nitika Sharma K. Gururaj, A.K. Mishra, RVS Pawaiya

ICAR- Central Institute for Research on Goats, Makhdoom, Mathura Uttar Pradesh

The livestock sector is a pillar of the global food system and a contributor to poverty reduction, food security and agricultural development. Livestock play a major role in sustainable food systems—for example, manure is a critical source of natural fertilizer, while livestock used as draft animals can help boost productivity in regions where there is low mechanization. Livestock are important assets for vulnerable communities.

Natural Animal Farming

Government of India is promoting natural farming, through National Mission on Natural Farming (NMNF) and organic farming through ParamparagatKrishiVikasYojna (PKVY) and Mission Organic Value Chain Development for North Eastern Region (MOVCDNER).On the initiative of NITI Ayog, Natural Farming defined as is a chemical-free traditional farming method. It is considered as an agroecology based diversified farming system which integrates crops, trees and livestock with functional biodiversity. Natural farming is a system where the laws of nature are applied to agricultural practices. This method works along with the natural biodiversity of each farmed area, encouraging the complexity of living organisms, both plants, and animals that shape each particular ecosystem to thrive along with food plants. Natural Farming builds on natural or ecological processes that exist in or around farms. Several studies have reported the effectiveness of natural farming in terms of increase in production, sustainability, saving of water use, improvement in soil health and farmland ecosystem. It is considered as a cost- effective farming practices with scope for raising employment and rural development. Natural Farming offers a solution to various problems, such as food insecurity, farmers' distress, and health problems arising due to pesticide and fertilizer residue in food and water, global warming, climate change and natural calamities. It also has the potential to generate employment, thereby stemming the migration of rural youth

Traditional Veterinary Medicine

The tradition medicines are in record to manage the clinical condition in animal and become the source of new drug formulation. The use of Ethno medicines or traditional medicine and medicinal plants in most developing countries for the maintenance of good health has been widely observed. Natural products have been the source of most active ingredients. This is widely accepted to be true when applied to drug discovery. More than 80% of drug substances invented in last decade were obtained from natural products or inspired by natural compounds. It is estimated that about 25% of the drugs prescribed worldwide are derived from plants and 121 such active compounds are in use. Of the total 252 drugs in WHO's essential medicine list, 11% is exclusively of plant origin. In India, about 80% of the rural population uses medicinal herbs or indigenous systems of medicine.

1. Ayurveda

Ayurveda originated in India long back in pre-vedic period. *Rigveda*and *Atharva-veda*(5000 years B.C.), the earliest documented ancient Indian knowledge have references on health and diseases. Ayurved texts like *CharakSamhita* and *SushrutaSamhita* were documented about 1000 years B.C. The term *Ayurveda* means 'Science of Life'. It deals elaborately with measures for healthful living during the entire span of life and its various phases. Besides, dealing with principles for maintenance of health, it has also developed a wide range of therapeutic measures to combat illness. These principles of positive health and therapeutic measures relate to physical, mental, social and spiritual welfare of human beings. Thus *Ayurveda* becomes one of the oldest systems of health care dealing with both the preventive and curative aspects of life in a most comprehensive way and presents a close similarity to the WHO's concept of health propounded in the modern era.

In human being ayurveda have, eight disciplines are generally called "Ashtanga Ayurveda" and are; Internal Medicine (*Kaya Chikitsa*), Paediatrics(*KaumarBhritya*), Psychiatry (*BhootVidya*), Otorhinolaryngology and Ophthalmology (*Shalakya*), Surgery(*Shalya*), Toxicology (*AgadTantra*), Geriatrics(*Rasayana*), Eugenics and aphrodisiacs(*Vajikarana*). Compendia on these subjects like *Charak Samihta, Sushruta Samhita* etc. were written by the ancient scholars during B.C. period. These were used for teaching of Ayurveda in the ancient universities of *Takshashila* and *Nalanda.* Basic theme of ayurvedatreatment consists of restoring the balance of disturbed body-mind matrix through regulating diet, correcting life-routine and behaviour, administration of drugs and resorting to preventive Panchkarma and *Rasayana* therapy.

There are two streams of practices; one is folk stream, comprising mostly the oral traditions practiced by the rural villages. The carriers of these traditions are millions of housewives, thousands of traditional birth attendants, bone setters, village practitioners skilled in acupressure, eye treatments, treatment of snake bites and the traditional village physicians/herbal healers, the vaidyas' or the tribal physicians. This stream of inherited traditions is together known as Local Health Traditions (LHT). At the second level of traditional health care system are the scientific or classical systems of medicine. This comprises of the codified and organized medicinal wisdom with sophisticated theoretical foundations and philosophical explanations expressed in classical texts like `Charka Samhita', `Sushrutasamhita', 'Bhelasamhita', and hundreds of other treatises including some in the regional languages covering treaties of all branches of medicine and surgery. Systems like Ayurveda, Siddha, Unani, Amchi and Tibetan, etc. are practiced.

Indian medicine is not reflected merely in the treatment of human beings but other important dimensions like veterinary medicine are addressed in detail through these systems. This represents a whole new spectrum of knowledge and opportunity. This area has not been exploited at all. The definition of Ayurvedic medicines under the Drugs & Cosmetics Act includes veterinary medicines. There are several authentic books of Ayurveda dealing with veterinary medicines such as NakulSamhita, PalkapyaShastra, Go Ayurveda, Hasti Ayurveda, BajNama etc. Central Government will encourage two institutions in the 10th Plan for introducing courses and undertaking documentation of the classical books in various languages. Homoeopathy also has effective treatment for care of animals and a similar approach would be followed.

In veterinary practice, ayurvedic drugs are used by utilizing academic knowledge of basics of physiology, biochemistry and diseases manifestation and as per indication given on the products. Among ayurvedic drugs, medicinal plants continue to be an important therapeutic content in it. In many eastern cultures such as those of India, China and the Arab/Persian world this experience was systematically recorded and incorporated into regular system of medicine that refined and developed and became a part of the MateriaMedica of these countries. Ayurveda is much superior among organized ancient systems of medicine. From history we learn that in the ancient times India was known as a place of rich natural resources, knowledge, wisdom and scholarship.

2. Traditional Veterinary Medicine (Ethno Veterinary Medicine)

Historically , Right from the Mahabharatha times, veterinary medicine was practised in India and documented in Sanskrit scriptures and literature in vernacular languages. The information in Sanskrit scriptures like the 'AsvaVaidyaka by Nakula', 'Palakpya', 'Garuda Purana', 'Asvayur Veda Sarasindu by Vysampayana', and 'Asvayur Veda Sara Sindhu by Malldeva' is well classified and documented according to the principles of the humoral theory of the Ayurvedic system. A few vernacular scriptures like 'SahadevaPasuVaidyaSastramu' (Telugu) and 'MattuVaidyaBodhini' (Tamil) are dealing with traditional veterinary medicine. Apart from the above, hundreds of references on treating animals with the locally available plant resources can be traced in vernacular articles which do not have the authenticity and authorship of the literature. Furthermore, numerous undocumented veterinary practices are in vogue in rural areas of India. Although Ayurvedic veterinary treatments are well documented in various Sanskrit scriptures, language barriers prevent their effective use.

Today we find a renewed interest in traditional medicine. During the past decade there have been an ever-increasing demand especially from developed countries for more and more drugs from plant sources. This revival of interest in plant-derived drugs is mainly due to the current widespread belief that `green medicine' is safe and more dependable than the costly synthetic drug many of which have adverse side effects. This resurgence of interest in the plant based drugs have necessitated an increased demand of medicinal plants leading to over-exploitation, unsustainable harvesting and finally to the virtual decimation of several valuable plant species in the wild. Moreover, the habitat degradation due to increased human activities (human settlements, agriculture and other developmental programmes, illegal trade in rare and endangered medicinal plants, and loss of regeneration potential of the degraded forests have further accelerated the current rate of extinction of plants particularly the medicinal plants.

In remote areas , livestock owners practiced traditional treatments because of no side effects ,Low costs and lack of modern veterinary facilities.

The diseases and conditions commonly treated with EVM included mastitis, fever, bloat, diarrhoea, and foot-and-mouth disease. Especially with husbandry-related problems such as mastitis, farmers believed that no external expertise was necessary but that they could manage treating these ailments with EVM. But the level of effectiveness of the treatment depended on the stage and severity of the disease. Nearly all farmers and traditional healers regarded fever as a disease. In general, in India, the commercialisation of herbal medicines may be connected with the long tradition of Ayurvedic medicine in this country. Ayurvedic scripts contain information on many plants and are often cited as an indication for the efficacy of these plants. Still, commercialized herbal medicine may be expensive for smallholders, especially when compared to self-made drugs . And if commercial herbal drugs are exported to other countries, they may there become nearly as expensive as other imported allopathic drugs. Unfortunately, there is little information on the economics of commercialized herbal drugs versus ethnoveterinary remedies prepared from scratch at the field level.

In India, ethnomedico-botanical surveys and inventories receive little attention and detailed information and documentation on the uses of medicinal plants in indigenous communities are lacking. This disinterest in the existing knowledge and neglect by authorities and public slowly result in the loss of this knowledge. It is high time that effective measures and programmes are adopted to save this information before it is lost forever. Ethnomedico-botanical surveys in each district are needed. Comparing and crosschecking the results will provide us with information about herbal medicines presently in use. Furthermore, concerted efforts are needed towards the usage of plant resources, linking conservation strongly with utilization.

ICAR effort in Documentation and Validation of Indigenous Technical Knowledge (ITK)

To prepare a package of simple, effective traditional veterinary treatments for rural India and require to validate treatments on an empirical basis by keeping quantitative and qualitative records of cases and their treatments. Documenting and validating ethnoveterinary practices are a first step towards preserving and promoting them. ICAR New Delhi, under a Net work project (NATP) on collection and documentation of Indigenous technical knowledge in the field of treatment of animals and subsequently their scientific validation to find out potential ITKs for their use by farmers and drug development by pharmaceutical Industry . As a result, Inventory have been prepared and published for scientist of the country. The four volumes has been published by ICAR. The ITKs were collected in agriculture and veterinary Practices

CIRG Herbal Technologies for Diseases Management

CIRG has developed herbal formulation as crude powder based or extract based or feed mix based in managing infection to maintain the production with non-chemical treatment approach. The main areas were identified as antistressor, immunomodulators ,anthelmintics, ectoparasites infestation , weaning stress, thermal stress and brucella Infection.

a. **Stressol powder for Ameliorating heat and cold stress:** The preparation for combating thermal stress was developed by a three plant extracts in suitable vehicle. The antioxidant efficacy of extract was tested under invitro by estimating free radicle scavenging, Lipid peroxidation etc. The clinical efficacy of this formulation was evaluated in heat stress, cold stress animals by monitoring stress markers in goats such as SOP, MDA, heat & cold and HSP 70 catalase. The formulation is effective in ameliorating the stress and positive effect on growth and production.

b. **Anti diarrhoeal preparation:** It is an extract base herbal anti-bacterial anti-diarrhoeal powder for management of diarrhea in animals. This herbal powder comprises the extracts of three plants with the additives effect to each other. Antibacterial efficacy was studied on Escherichia coli, most prevalent entero- pathogens. Antibacterial, parasympatholytic, astringent activity results to control the diarrhoea in goats .

c. **The topical antiseptic gel:** This formulation is used to treat skin infection including the septic wound and maggot wound.

d. **Anthelmintic formulation:** Anthelimintic resistance against internal parasite is growing problem. Herbal drug is effective alternate in treatment. This herbal bolus contains active ingredients of three medicinal plants. Herbal formulation tested under invitroagaint Adult worm, larval stage and egg and additive effect. This bolus is given at the schedule of one daily for 2-3 days and reduces the EPG by 60-70 percent. It mainly tested against the Haemonchuscontortus infection in goat . This can be given as bolus or feed mix to control the parasite and useful for organic farming

e. **Herbal immunomodulatory bolus**: This herbal formulation developed to improve immunity in pregnant goat and colostral immunity, thus improve the passive immunity in born kid to fight against neonatal infection. This bolus reduces the cortisol level, improve the immunoglobulin in pregnant dam in given schedule. Colostral IgG and IgM values increased. In born kids , and serum IgG, IgM , protein levels increased and effectively managed E coli LPS administration experiment. This is valuable as bolus /feed mix in pregnant stage. Reccommended in schedule of 5 gram one bolus daily for 3-4 week period in goats

f. **Herbal acaricidal liquid /spray:** The Ticks and lice management in animals by synthetic chemical poses the resistance and herbal therapy is effective acceptable alternate. Formulation contains extract of two or three medicinal plants in two preparations selected on the basis of lowest LC 50, LC 90 values, mortality at 24 hrs, lowest Estimated reproduction factor and highest Inhibition reproduction %. This formulation effectively eiliminate 90-100% ticks in single topical application. This can be used as water soluble or spray.

g. **Aja-Sanjeevani-Herbal Immunomodulatory Formulation for Amelioration of Weaning Stress in Goat kids:** Aja- Sanjeevani is a herbal immunomodulatory formulation for the amelioration of weaning stress which was standardized and validated in weaned kids of Barbari. It ameliorates the post-weaning stress resulting in reduced post-weaning mortality and morbidity, better body weight gain and thus increased profits from goat-farming. It is a non-antibiotic intervention will result in clean and organic chevon production. It is herbal immunomodulatory ameliorates the weaning stress and increase the survivability of goat kids at the time of weaning by reducing the post weaning morbidity and mortality. Aja-Sanjeevani is – easy to admister, effective, economical and non-antibiotic formulation.

h. **EASY KIDDER"- a herbal formula to minimize parturition problems:** This formulation will optimize the oxidative stress and inflammation in dam as well as the kid , and thereby promote the tissue growth and repair in goat thus , increase productivity in terms of higher body weight gain of kids and increased milk production in dam along with reduced disease incidence. This is formulated into bolus (5gm herbal mixture per bolus) with help of bidder/excipients.Pregnant animals fed one bolus each for 15 days before expected.

i. **Brucare herbal powder for checking brucella organism:** This is herbal product in the form of Bolus was developed to reduce shedding of Brucella and it was found to contain the spread of infection in small ruminants. This organism causes abortion in goat and potentially zoonotic.

j. **Herbal anticoccidial complete pellet feed formulation for goats:** Medicated complete feed containing herbal anticoccidial ingredients, provide all the nutrient required by the goat and also help in reducing the effect of coccidia infection. This feed will improve the production performance during the critical age of goats without the use of chemical anticoccidial drug. This is also consumer friendly technology as the goat consuming this feed will produce healthy goat products with no drug or chemical residue. Improvement in body weight gain and daily dry matter intake (g) in goats were recorded. Production parameters affected due to coccidial infection get improved by feeding of pellet containing herbal anticoccidial feed mix.

k. **Low Methane producing Herbal complete pellet feed for goats:** In India contribution of goat in methane emission through enteric fermentation was 4.7 % in total methane production from livestock. This feed formulation will provide the entire nutrient required by the animals. Average body weight gain per day by feeding of this feed was 70.98 gram in barbari goats. This complete pellet feed formulation produced 20.04% less methane on per day basis and 19.69% less methane on dry matter intake basis. The pellet feed is free from chemical additive, making it a consumer friendly technology. Feeding of this feed will not have any harmful residue in goat products.

l. **Phage based oral therapy for neonatal diarrhoea:** The cocktail mixture of phages against E coli found effective in controlling theneonatal diarrhoea , reducing the use of chemical antibacterial drugs

Natural livestock farming reduces cost of supplements and antibiotics and other chemicals, which in turn producing products free from antibiotic and chemical residue.

References

Anjara, J. 1996 Ethnoveterinary Pharmacology in India: Past, Present and Future. In: Ethnoveterinary Research and Development. eds. McCorkle, C.M., Mathias, E. and chillhorn van veen, T.W., Intermediate Technology Publications, London, UK, pgs. 137 – 147.

Beasler DE and Kroening , R J 1976 *Three essential factors in effective acupuncture therapy* (Fide : Schoen, AM and Wynn S G (1997) *Complementary and alternative veterinary Medicine* . Mosby, St loius)

World Bank 1997. *Medicinal Plants – Rescuing a Global Heritage*. eds. Lambert, J., Srivastava, J. and Vietmeyer, N., Technical Paper No. 355, pgs. 61.

Duke Wain, 1981 (Medicinal plants of the world ,) are available on internet (http:// www.ars-grin.gov/~ngrlsb

ICAR Inventory of Indigenous Technical Knowledge in Agriculture documents 1, 2 ,3 (NATP) ICAR publication.

Bhat, K K S 1997. Medicinal and plant information databases. In: *Medicinal Plants for Forests Conservation and Health Care*. eds. Bodeker, G. and Vantomne, P.,FAO, Non-Wood Forest Products Series No. 11, FAO, Rome, pgs. 158.

7

Organic Livestock Production Standards and Certification Procedures in India

P Baswa Reddy

Principal Scientist, ICAR-National Meat Research Institute, Hyderabad Telangana

With increasing demand from consumers for organically produced and certified food products in the country, organic agriculturein India is growing steadily as more and more farmers are adopting organic practices to meet the increasing demand.. Starting with organic tea and spices, it's grown to organic flour, breakfast cereals, fruits, vegetables and many more, the number of food categories sold as organic is growing rapidly in India. Of late, the consumer demand for organically produced livestock products like milk, eggs and meat is also on the rise.

Domestic organic food products market in India is witnessing a growth rate of around 20% CAGR in the recent years. The COVID-19 pandemic has also led to consumer awareness about the quality of foods and contributed to the growth of organic food market in the country. As a result, informal markets for organic products are getting established to serve the niche consumers and simultaneously, producer to consumer market is also gaining momentum. Local markets are also now vending perishable organic foods like fruits and vegetables. During 2020-21 in India, there were around 16 lakh organic producers under NPOP production system producing 34.9 lakh tons of organic products in 43.3 lakh hectares of land including 16.8 lakh hectares under wild harvest. During this period, 8.88 lakh tons of organic products worth Rs.7078 crores were exported from India. Under Participatory Guaranty System (PGS) in India, as of September 2021, there are about 42 thousand organic farmer groups comprising of around 12 lakh farmers producing organic products in 75 lakh hectares of land. Madhya Pradesh, Maharashtra, Karnataka, Rajasthan and Uttar Pradesh are the major organic production states in the country and the major commodities produced are oil seeds, fibre, sugar, cereals, millets, spices and condiments. USA, EU, Canada and Australia are major export destinations of Indian organic products and the major organic products exported from India are processed foods, oil seeds, cereals, millets, spices and tea.

Though organic crop production and certification system is reasonably well established in India, the organic livestock and poultry sector is in its budding stage. Organizations such as APEDA, FSSAI and BIS along with research establishments like ICAR- National Meat Research Institute are now putting serious efforts to establish the protocols and promote organic livestock production and certification in India. As a result, in the last few years, livestock farmers are gradually getting encouraged to take up organic production and around 3000 farmers mostly from Uttar Pradesh, Madhya Pradesh and Himachal Pradesh have taken up organic dairy, sheep and poultry farming. Export of organic milk and ghee from India to different countries has just begun and is expected to grow very fast in volumes and revenues in the years to come.

Organic Meat and Milk Production

Organic livestock production and marketing of organic livestock products like milk, meat and eggs have witnessed an upward trend in growth rate worldwide in the last decade. In 2020 the organic dairy market crossed the USD 20 billion and as per the estimates of market experts, it is expected to reach USD 32 billion by 2026 with CAGR of more than 6%. In India, organic milk market is still in its infancy and it was worth Rs 450 crores in 2020 and the market analysts expect it to grow at more than 30% CAGR up to 2026.

The global organic meat products market is expected grow from USD 15 billion in 2020 to USD 20 billion in 2025 at a CAGR of around 7%. In India, the organic meat sector is yet to take off. A few organic sheep, poultry and pig units have recently been established and the certified organic meat from these units is likely enter the markets in the next one or two years. Since India already occupies number one position in buffalo meat export in the world, using these established channels for male buffalo calf rearing on organic lines and exporting such organic meat has the potential to keep India in a prominent position in world organic meat map.

As conventional livestock production practices are frequently criticized in the context of food safety concerns and animal disease outbreaks, there is growing consumer demand to move away from the widespread use of antibiotics and feed additives and to strengthen animal welfare standards. With increasing concern for animal welfare and environmental preservation consumers are now looking for alternative livestock production systems, which follow natural process of animal production with utmost regards for food safety and food security. This has led to the concept of organic meat, egg and milk consumption by the public. Organic animal production system is emerging as an effective alternative to address all these issues. Owing to this, in India, there are bright prospects for tapping this opportunity to develop it into a business model in Animal Husbandry sector. However, among many other issues, the profitability of organic livestock and poultry farming *vis a vis* conventional farming, is the crucial one from the point of view of the Indian farmers, particularly the small and marginal.

Organic Livestock and Poultry Production Standards

The broad guidelines for organic livestock production under National Programme for Organic Production (NPOP) of India are as under:

Organic management plan: Before starting organic livestock farming, producer has to make a detailed organic management plan and present it to the certifying agency for approval.

Breed /Strain selection: Local breeds / strains which can easily be acclimatized to local climatic conditions shall be preferred over the exotic breeds

Source / Origin: Initial stock should be sourced from organically certified units. If the animals are introduced from non-organic units, they should undergo mandatory conversion period as specified for each category of livestock/ poultry.

Housing and management: Livestock and poultry shall be maintained under natural conditions as far as possible. This shall include utilizing natural breeding methods, housing and management conditions tominimize stress, health management system to prevent diseases. Minimum shaded as well as open area as specified for each category of livestock / poultry shall be followed.

Conversion period: Animals brought from non-organic sources shall undergo conversion period as specified for each category of livestock and poultry. During the conversion period the animals should be maintained under organic conditions. After completion of conversion period, the animals can be sold as organic.

Feeding: Livestock and poultry shall be provided with organically produced feed during the entire rearing period. The agriculture land committed for cultivation of feed / fodder crops intended to be used as feed for livestock and poultry shall be organic. The overall feeding practices shall satisfy the daily nutrient requirements of the concerned animals.

Feed additives and supplements used for feeding shall be from natural sources and as permitted under organic livestock guidelines.

Healthcare: The organic livestock & poultry, in general, should follow the basic principles of preventive health and productivity management wherein the focus would be on preventing diseases, detecting underlying fertility and production problems and its correction primarily on correcting management, nutrition and sanitation. Antibiotics and other allopathic drugs are not permitted. For purpose of treatment and prevention of diseases and under-performances, herbal/ phyto-therapeutic (excluding antibiotics), homeopathic or ayurvedic products shall be preferred to allopathic veterinary drugs or antibiotics, provided that their therapeutic effect is effective for the species of animal and the condition for which the treatment is intended.Antibiotic and other allopathic drugs can be used when other modes of cure are not effective to save the life of the animal and in such cases withdrawal periods as prescribed for each drug should be strictly followed. Hormonal treatment and use of growth promotors shall not be permitted. All vaccinations required by law of the land shall be permitted.

Breeding and Management: The preference for reproduction shall be through natural methods, although artificial insemination may be used. Embryo transfer techniques and the use of hormonal reproductive treatment shall not be used unless prescribed for therapeutic purpose directed towards correcting the physiological problem. The breeding techniques employing genetic engineering shall not be used.

Manure and urine management: Manure and urine excreta collection and management practices in the organic livestock & poultry farm are a critical component. The collection, handling and disposal of the dung and

urine from shed, paddock, open run or grazing areas shall be implemented in a manner that minimizes soil and water degradation, does not significantly contribute to contamination of water, optimizes recycling of nutrients and does not include burning or any practice inconsistent with organic practices.

Transport: During transport, the producer shall prevent stress, injury, hunger, thirst, malnutrition, fear,distress, physical & thermal discomfort, pain, diseaseduring the transport and shall observe all the conditions set in law of the land for animal transportation. Animals must be fit for the intended journey. All necessary arrangement shall be made in advance to minimize length of the journey and meet the animal's need during the journey. Means of transport as well as the loading and unloading facilities must be designed, constructed, maintained and operated so as to avoid injury and suffering and ensure the safety of the animals.

Slaughter: The slaughter of livestock and poultry shall be undertaken in a manner, which minimizes stress and suffering, and shall be in accordance with the territorial/ national rules framed for the purpose. Minimum age of slaughter for each species of livestock should be followed as prescribed for the respective species.

Organic Livestock Certification

Production of crops or livestock like sheep and goats organically without validation or auditing has limited reach to the consumers. The consumers of organic products cannot always verify the production practices followed by the organic producers and hence they need authenticity to rely upon. Certification of organic products and processes serves this purpose and improves the consumer confidence and there by widens the market for the organic produce.

In India, there are different avenues available for certification of organic produce. Each system of certification has its own purpose, merits and constraints. Farmers interested in organic farming need to assess the pros and cons in each system of certification and choose the one which fulfils their requirement.

The different avenues of organic certification in India are

3. NPOP certification
4. Participatory Guarantee System (PGS)

The NPOP (National Programme for Organic Production) certification system of India involves a third party inspection to ascertain the compliance of organic production system. The certification is supervised by the APEDA at national level. APEDA authorizes the eligible certification agencies through a process of accreditation and these certification bodies can take up the certification at farm/ producer/ processor/ grower group level. Certification process is carried out as per the laid down standards and guidelines of organic livestock and poultry production. The produce certified under NPOP is entitled to carry the 'India Organic' logo along with 'Jaivik Bharat' logo as specified by FSSAI and can be sold within India and also can be exported to other countries as organic product after complying with the requirements of the importer.

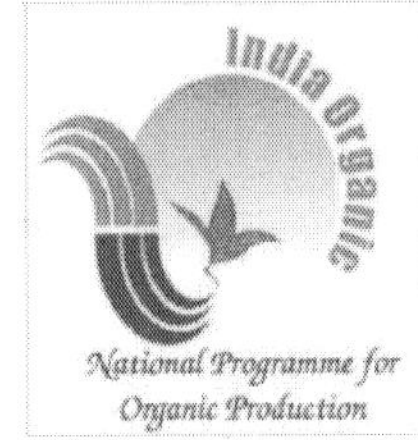

Participatory Guarantee System (PGS) is a quality assurance initiative that is locally relevant, emphasize the participation of stakeholders, including producers and consumers and operate outside the frame of third party certification. This certification is based on active participation of stakeholders and is built on a foundation of trust, social networks and knowledge exchange. It is for farmers or communities that can organize and perform as a group within the village or in close-by villages with continuous territory. PGS ensures traceability only up to end till it is in the custody of the group. Once the product leaves the custody of PGS group there is no control of PGS on its integrity. The produce certified under PGS can use the logo of 'PGS- Green' (for farm/ produce under conversion) or 'PGS- Organic' (for farm/ produce completely concerted to Organic) along with Jaivik Bharat logo as specified by FSSAI and can be sold within India as organic product.

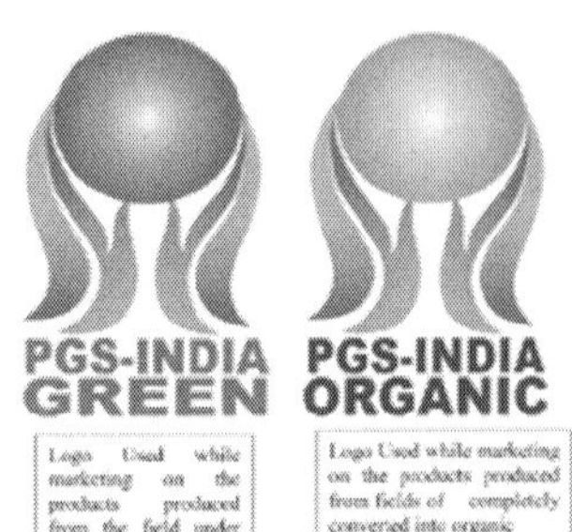

Certified organic fodder production or certification of grazing land is in similar lines to the certification of crops which is fairy established in India.Organic certification of livestock products (value added products of meat, milk etc.,) is considered in the similar category as that of certification of processed foods and other value added food products which requires organic processing certification.

The process of becoming organically certified can be expensive, but it is an essential step for farmers and manufacturers wanting to meet the growing demand for certified organic food among the quality conscious consumers which fetches premium price for their produce.

Promotion of Organic Production by the Government

The Government of India has introduced multiple schemes and incentives to encourage the adoption of organic farming by the farmers. The most prominent schemes of the government for promotion of organic farming in India areParamparagat Krishi Vikas Yojana (PKVY), Mission Organic Value Chain Development in NE Region (MOVCDNER) National Project on Organic Farming(NPOF), Rashtriya Krishi Vikas Yojana (RKVY), Mission for Integrated Development of Horticulture (MIDH), ICAR-Network Project on Organic farming, NamamiGange Project etc.,

Paramparagat Krishi Vikas Yojana (PKVY) is an elaborated component of Soil Health Management (SHM) of major project National Mission of Sustainable Agriculture (NMSA). Under PKVY Organic farming is promoted through adoption of organic village by cluster approach and PGS certification. The Scheme envisagesPromotion of commercial organic production through certified organic farming. Groups of farmers are encouraged to take up organic farming under PKVY and they are motivated for natural resource mobilization for input production. There will be no liability on the farmers for expenditure on certification. Every farmer will be provided with some monitory support on per acre basis for three years. Organic farming will be promoted by using traditional resources and the organic products will be linked with the market.

Challenges

Certification of both fodder and livestock: Unlike organic crop certification where a producer is required to get his only the concerned crop certified, a farmer who wishes to take up organic small ruminant production needs to obtain certification for both fodder as well as the animals. Thus it requires double certification compliances in case of organic small ruminant production.

Awareness: Lack of awareness among the farmers about the guidelines of organic livestock & poultry farming and the processes available for their certification is the main hurdle hindering the development of this sector in the country.

Non availability of certified feed and fodder: Lack of availability of organically certified feed in the market is a major setback for the beginners till they establish their own certified feed and fodder production unit to meet the feed requirements of the livestock unit.

Lack of awareness on Ethno-veterinary Medicine: Since organic livestock production does not permit usage of synthetic products like antibiotics and hormones for animal health care, it entirely relies on traditional systems of medicine like ethno-veterinary medicine (EVM) for animal healthcare. However, not many veterinarians in the country have expertise in EVM procedures for animal healthcare and this system of health care for various disease conditions of animals needs to be standardized and popularized in the country to effectively take care of animals under organic production.

Certification: Very few organic certifying agencies in India have accreditation for livestock certification. In case of organic crop certification under PGS, in many states, the machinery of state agricultural departments is involved in organic certification but the same is lacking in case of livestock certification.

Labour: Currently, organic food production is assumed to be more labour intensive since under this system the farmers are advised to be more animal welfare friendly and adopt traditional health care systems which involves relatively higher labour when compared to allopathic health care.

Documentation: Documentation of all the processes and activities in organic production and marketing of the produce like under NPOP system is a cumbersome process for an ordinary farmer

Productivity: Initially, the productivity of organic livestock farms is likely to be lower than the traditional commercial farms till the organic livestock management, nutrition, health care and reproduction practices are fine tuned for higher productive yields.

Costs: Organic certification is expensive and organic feed for animals can cost twice that of normal feed. Organic farms tend to be smaller than conventional farms, which means fixed costs and overhead must be distributed across smaller produce volumes without government subsidies.

*Market:*Organised market for organic livestock products is yet to evolve in the country. Since there is no stringent enforcement mechanism, the certified organic produce has to face competition from non-certified and dubious produce sold in the market.

However, as the markets for organic products get matured and certified organic livestock products gain consumer confidence, these products fetch premium price which can nullifying the higher costs involved in production and certification.

Prospects and Entrepreneurial Opportunities

Since organic livestock rearing and organic livestock products preparation are yet to take a leap in India, there are possibilities of entrepreneurial opportunities in all spheres of organic value chain right from production through certification, value addition, marketing till consumption. All the products and services in the organic food value chain are likely to fetch premium price in the market as they are targeted for niche consumers who are quality conscious and would be willing to pay premium price for quality products.

India already occupies number one position in buffalo meat export in the world. This can be potentially extended to organic meat production by rearing male buffalo calves on organic lines to export certified organic buffalo meat and put India in a prominent position in world organic meat map.

Certified organic feed and fodder is a crucial input for organic livestock rearing. Some farmers can produce certified organic feed and fodder and supply it to organic livestock producers. Those who have resources may produce and market both organic fodder and livestock as well. This sector also throws huge opportunities for veterinarians who specialize in traditional and ethnoveterinary practices of animal health care. Other opportunities in organic livestock value chain include certification agencies, inspection executives, Organic livestock production process advisors, organic product quality testing, organic products preparation like meat & milk products, wholesale and retail marketing, establishment of organic meat & milk outlets and export of organic meat, milk, eggs etc.,

However, despite the growing interest in organic livestock production, it still faces several challenges, including a lack of awareness among producers about the production standards and certification process, lack of proper infrastructure, high production costs, and limited marketing opportunities. Nonetheless, the government's continued support for organic farming and livestock production, combined with increasing consumer demand for organic products, is expected to drive the growth of the sector in the coming years.

8

Goat Milk Products Market Potential in India and Abroad

Arpita Nag

Meraki Artisan Cheeseand Rustic Bakes, Kolkata, West Bengal

Our nation happens to be the largest producer of goat milk globally and it is high time that we use this to our advantage. India happens to be one of the fastest growing economies of the world and the IMF projects our GDP is set to rise at a healthy rate of 5.9 % in 2023, the highest among all other economies.

Goat Production in Field Conditions

We are an agro-based nation with 70% of our population residing in rural areas. As we deliberate today on the best possible ways to facilitate natural goat farming, we have to remember that such traditional agrarian practices is the essence of our Indian ethos, from ancient times. Such wisdom has been passed on for generations and it is great to witness that the world is waking up to the benefits of the natural versus the synthetic be it in clothing or food or lifestyle in general.

Goats have been dubbed as "poor man's cows" owing to their low maintenance and easy adaptability to harsh climactic conditions. They are reared by marginal farmers and nomadic pastoral communities across various parts of our country. They can be naturally grazed on public pastures and forest lands and hence do not form a source of burden for their owners. Apart from the logistical and financial benefit, let us also understand that free grazing cattle gives the best quality milk in terms of taste, texture and nutrition. As a natural cheesemaker I have had the experience of working with various types of milk – organic, raw, pasteurized, free grazing cattle milk, milk from stall fed cattle and the most important observation that I can make is that raw milk obtained from free grazing cows or goats or buffaloes produce the best quality cheese. This happens due to various factors.

There is a word "terroir" that is frequently used in the wine industry. It means the characteristic taste and flavour imparted to a wine by the environment in which it is produced. Similarly, the natural or artisan cheese making industry across the world is dependent on the terroir of the milk to produce the best quality cheeses. And this natural environment in which the cattle if grazing imparts the cheese its characteristic flavour, taste, texture thus making each type of cheese unique as per its geographical location. And to protect this uniqueness, various areas of different countries have PDO (Protected Designation of Origin) cheeses much like our GI tags. So for example Greek feta can only be made in Greece and the world famous Parmesan or parmigiano reggiano cheese can only be produced in a few provinces in northern Italy. There are many such cheeses across the world that have such protection in order to prevent imitation.

Now let us understand why it is so important to demarcate cheeses as per the geographical location. The answer is terroir again. Natural cheese making depends on the microbial activity that takes place in naturally grazed cattle milk. Cheese making is essentially the process of letting the naturally occurring bacteria, fungi and yeasts develop in their micro habitat. And each of these micro habitats depend on the flora and fauna of a particular place in which a particular cattle is grazing. As a result just as a British cheese maker will not be able to develop a cheese that is originally made in a particular region of France, if we try to make cheese from milk of goats grazing in the Himalayan meadows and those in the arid areas of Rajasthan the resultant products will be very different from one another and distinctly unique in their own way.

Thus natural goat rearing in field conditions produces the ideal quality of milk for natural cheese making.

Goat Milk – Benefits and Uses

As an artisan cheesemaker I often get asked about the benefits of goat cheese in comparison to cow milk/ buffalo milk cheeses. The benefits of goat milk are multiple. Some of them are as follows:

1. It is lower in lactose, so can be digested by lactose intolerant people.
2. It is packed with minerals like that calcium, phosphorus, copper, magnesium & selenium. It is also high in Vitamin A & B3 and Omega 3 fatty acid.
3. Goat milk has lower fat globules in comparison to cow milk and is therefore easier to digest
4. The fat molecules are made of medium chain fatty acids which break down easily with digestion. This helps in quick release of energy thus making it more filling than cow cheese. Consequently we eat lesser.

Thus goat cheese can actually help in weight loss. About 28g is the ideal daily intake for chevre or any other type of goat cheese.

5. Goat milk is known for its antibacterial properties & is therefore prescribed as antidote to quite a few ailments, in traditional medicine
6. It is higher in A2 protein (that has lesser allergen) compared to A1 milk & therefore causes less inflammation of our stomach
7. It contains high levels probiotic that promotes good bacteria in the gut

All these factors are important when we are dealing with the various uses to which goat milk can be put to. Some of the products made from goat milk that can be listed as beneficial for human consumption are

Goat Milk
Butter
Ghee
Paneer
Cheese
Yoghurt
Powdered Milk
Formula Milk
Soap

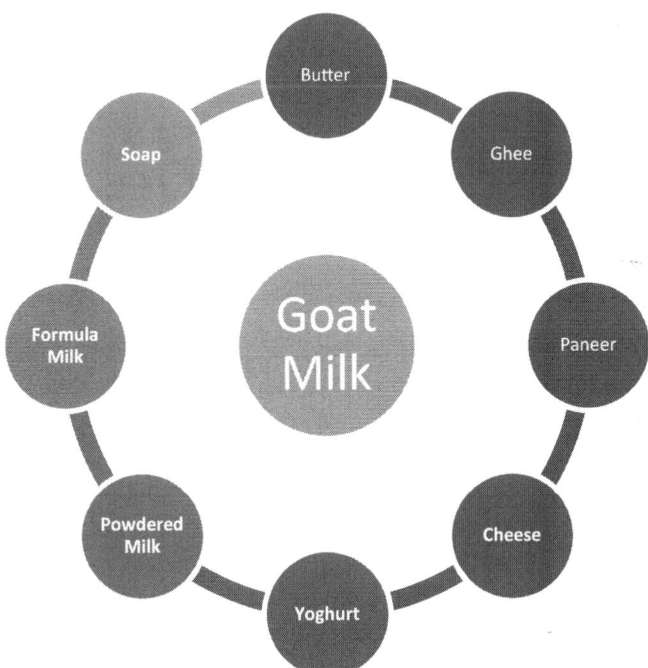

A Rajasthan based company by the name of Aadvik Foods was recently funded by Shark Tank India for their innovative dairy based products made out of goat and camel milk.

Domestic Market Potential

India is the largest producer of milk with a 23.67 percent share in total milk production in the world ot of which goat milk has a 3% share. However the lack of cooperatives/ organizations in most rural areas leave huge number of untapped resources. A lot of surplus milk go for a waste since there are no takers in such areas. And even in places where there are milk cooperatives, cattle rearing for milk does not seem to be a very lucrative option, since the price of milk received by cattle herders is minimal.

Urban consumers on the hand, have limited access to fresh, unadulterated milk/ milk products. Dairy products, in this case **cheese** can serve as a good solution to this problem by bridging the gap between the rural resource surplus and the unmet urban demand.

Artisan cheese is handmade cheese made with no or minimum machine intervention and without any artificial enhancer or preservatives. All the goodness of milk remains intact in such cheese and can be consumed as one of the richest sources of protein in one's diet.

From the market point of view, there is definitely a high demand for artisan cheese. People these days are conscious of what goes on their plate and the place from where it is sourced. Hence the 'vocal for local' concept too has been gaining momentum. People are realizing that it is way healthier to consume locally grown/ produced food items in comparison to fancy store bought, chemically preserved, mass market, factory produced counterparts. And with the internet opening up a world of global cuisine, people are ready to experiment more and try out products like cheese for everyday and gourmet cooking.

Goat cheese is a niche product and is hence expensive. The yield of milk from indigenous breeds is quite less in comparison to say a Sanen or an Alpine breed. And as a result the availability of milk is not as easy as that of cow's milk. And there is a gap when it comes to getting access to this milk for various milk based products. While the skill set required to make such products lies with a few, the inability to access good quality milk in urban settings becomes the biggest challenge for an urban cheese making company like ours and other artisan cheese making companies in India. The market for goat cheese in India is gradually growing. Given the taste profile of the cheese with its tangy and earthy smell it has got a slower acceptance rate in comparison to more popular cow milk cheeses like a mozzarella or gouda or cheddar. However well-travelled Indians have a greater taste for such cheeses and are gradually shifting to domestically made cheeses as opposed to imported varieties. Five star hotels and restaurants are regularly experimenting with new varieties of cheeses and are regular customers of such products, also because of their inflow of international guests.

Export Potential

Internationally, the growth potential of the goat cheese market is projected at a highly accelerated rate. While countries in Asia and Africa happen to be the largest consumers of goat milk, North America followed by Europe is set to lead the market followed by the Asia Pacific when it comes to consumption of goat cheeses. Traditionally France has been and is the largest producer of goat milk cheeses both in terms of volume and variety, followed by other European and North American countries.

The Goat Cheese Market is Expected to Reach the Value of USD 14.66 Billion by 2029

(*Data Bridge Market Research)

Following is the list of countries in order of market share of goat cheese consumption

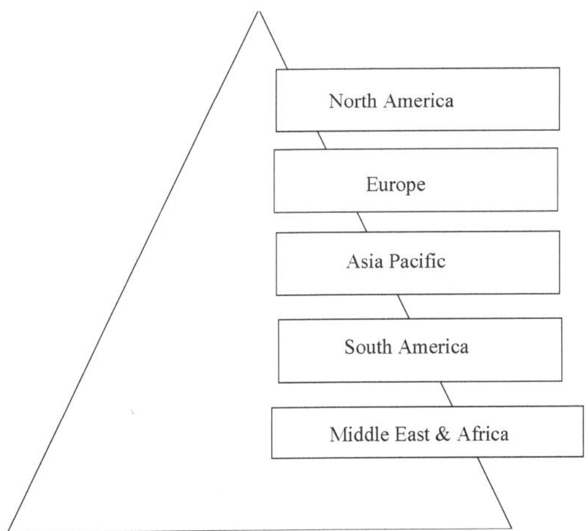

Goat Cheese Market Analysis

"The Goat Cheese market is projected to register a CAGR of 5.3% during the forecast period, 2022-2029.

Widespread acceptance of goat cheese in several countries owing to its health benefits is the primary driver of the market. Additionally, goat cheese producers are introducing goat cheese in different flavours in response to consumers' rising interest in fresh, healthful dairy products. For instance, goat cheese is preferred over its conventional counterparts as it contains more protein and less cholesterol than cow cheese. Moreover, the market is being driven by improvements in goat breed quality and technological advancements in cheese production.

Europe is the world's top producer of goat cheese, with France serving as its largest market. Retail sales are anticipated to be driven by the rising demand for goat cheese products in developed economies including the United States, France, and Germany. Africa and Asia are among the regions that eat the most goat milk, although these regions consume less goat cheese than developed markets. However, the rising prevalence of obesity and cholesterol-related disorders in these regions is anticipated to stimulate the preference for goat cheese during the forecast period."

***Source: Goat Cheese Market – Growth, Trends, Covid-19 Impact, and Forecasts (2023 – 2028) by Mordor Intelligence**

Key Challenges

- Lack of awareness about the market potential of goat cheese since cheese is not an indigenous food product that we have grown up on
- Sourcing of good quality naturally grazed goat milk in abundance since the yield of cheese from milk is about 10%, meaning 10L of milk will produce 1Kg cheese, 100L will produce 1Kg
- Bridging the gap between cattle owners and their earning potential from a globally acclaimed milk product like cheese by providing the right kind of market linkage
- Cheese being a highly perishable product, the cold chain logistics is of utmost importance

Probable Solutions

- Creating awareness among goat owners/ farmers about the potential of goat milk products like cheese
- Extensive training in production, packaging, hygiene and quality control of such products
- Education on how to rear and care for cattle for utmost milk yield
- Creating market linkage at domestic followed by international levels
- Setting up and maintaining of high quality cold chain packaging and transport logistics

9

Organic Goat Produce Opportunities and Challenges

Vikas Pathak, Meena Goswami and Sanjay Kumar Bharti

Department of Livestock Products Technology College of Veterinary Science & Animal Husbandry, DUVASU, Mathura, Uttar Pradesh

India is bestowed with huge livestock population reared under diverse production systems and agro-climatic conditions. Livestock sector is great importance for the sustainability of rural economies and many ecosystems. The economic importance of livestock activity is reflected by the weight of the agricultural sector in the national gross domestic product. The share of livestock sector to the national GDP has increased more than 56% over the span of ten years to 6.17% in 2020-21 from 3.94% in 2010-11. The contribution of the livestock sector, mean while, to total agriculture GVA has increased to 30.87 per cent from 20 per cent during the corresponding period. The livestock sector employs about 8.8% of the population and provides livelihood to two third of rural communities in India.

India occupies first position in terms of goat population and milk production. Since ancient times goat milk has traditionally been known for its medicinal properties and has recently gained importance in human health due to its proximity to human milk for easy digestibility and it's all round health promoting traits. The goats are also important for chevon production; the most preferred and relished meat in India. As per 20th Livestock Census, the total population of goats in the country is estimated at 148.88 million numbers. Goat milk has continued to play an important role in human nutrition in the area acknowledged as the cradle of modern civilization (Hatziminaoglou and Boyazoglu, 2004). Goat milk is having better digestibility, alkalinity, buffering capacity and certain therapeutic values in medicine and human nutrition in comparison to cow's or human milk. Goat milk is considered the best milk for infants because of predominance of smaller fat globules causing faster lipase activity which results in easy digestibility of goat milk (Chandan et al.,1992). Goat milk also contains three characteristics fatty acids *i.e.* caproic acid, caprylic and capric acid which are having medicinal values for patients suffering from malabsorption, childhood epilepsy, cystic fibrosis and gallstones (Haenlin, 1992). Demand for goat milk and milk products for internal consumption and export is expected to rise in coming years. The global goat milk market size was valued at $8.5 billion in 2018, and is expected to reach $11.4 billion by 2026, growing at a CAGR of 3.8% from 2019 to 2026. The total milk production from goats in 2021-2021 was 6.46 million tones contributing about 2.93% of the total milk production across the country.

Goat meat is the healthiest meat among red meats known for human consumption. Nutritionally, goat meat is an important source of high quality proteins, healthy fats, with low calorie and intramuscular fat as well as good source of essential amino acids, namely leucine, isoleucine, lysine, methionine, phenylalanine, threonine, tryptophan and valine etc. Goat meat on average consists of 72.3% moisture, 21.0% protein, 4.7% fat and 1.1% ash per 100 g of fresh meat (Dhanda, 2001). The chevon production in 2021-2022 was 1.26 million tons accounting to 13.63% to the total meat production (BAHS, 2022). Besides meat production, the slaughter house by-products like hides/skins, bones, intestines, blood etc. are economically important for domestic as well as international trade. Pashmina is another valuable produce from goat which is softest, warmest and costliest woolen fabric. Due to the growing demand for animal products, there is a need to design new livestock production systems that allow the combination of food security and sustainability. There has been considerable growth in the number of organic livestock farms in response to the necessity to fulfill the growing demand for animal products predicted for 2050 (FAO, 2009). Therefore, researchers are primarily aimed at strengthening and diversification of commodity optimization of technological manufacturing, assortment of production in terms of nutritional value, innovation mode of presentation of products obtained from goats.

Organic Farming

The philosopher Rudolf Steiner founded biodynamic farming during a series of lectures given at an agricultural course in Germany in 1924. The term organic farming was first used by Lord Northboure in 1940.JI Rodale, popularized the term and methods of organic growing, particularly to consumers through promotion of organic gardening. In 1981, the organic farmers coordinated with international body called International Federation of Organic Agriculture Movements (IFOAM), which prepares guidelines for cultivation and processing. As per FAO, the organic farming is a special type of production management that uses on-farm agronomic, biological, and mechanical approaches instead of any artificial off-farm inputs to support and increase the health of agro-ecosystems, including biodiversity, biological cycles, and soil biological activities (Kulhade et al., 2016). As per the Codex Alimentarius commission guidelines, organic farming may be defined as "a holistic production management system, which promotes and enhances agro-ecosystem health including biodiversity, biological cycles and soil biological activity". The guidelines have also established principles of organic production from the stages of production, processing, storage and transport to labeling and marketing. Organic production is different from the conventional production mainly due to its stress on conserving the fertility of soil, avoiding pollution, producing food of optimum nutritional quality, minimizing the usage of non renewable resources, etc.

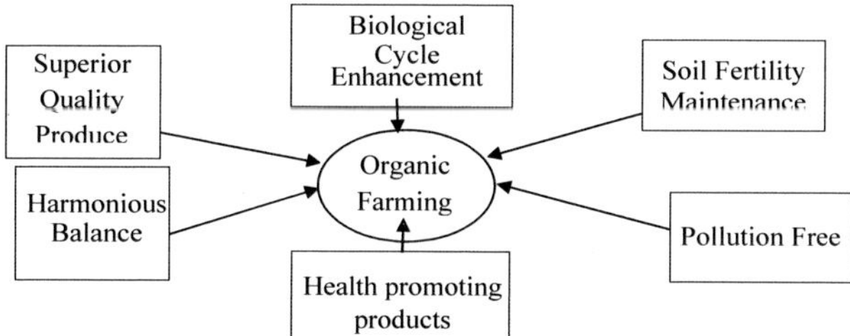

Objectives of Organic Farming

Organic farming is a growing business throughout the globe due to the growing demand for safe and healthy food and concerns about environmental pollution caused by indiscriminate application of agrochemicals. The preference towards health organic foods is expected to rise manifolds after emergence of COVID, a global deadly epidemic. The organic farming in India can be traced back to prehistoric times as narrated in Indian scriptures Ramayana, Rig-Veda, Mahabharata and many more (Bhattacharyya and Chakraborty, 2005). In the present times, organic agriculture is practiced in 187 countries managing about 72.3 million hectares. Land area for organic agricultural production is the largest in Australia followed by Argentina and Spain. As per the available statistics, India's rank 5thin terms of World's Organic Agricultural land and 1stin terms of total number of producers as per 2021 data (FIBL & IFOAM Year Book, 2020). The organic food export realization was around Rs. 5249.32 crore (771.96 million USD). India ranks first in Asia (fifth in the world) with 23 lakh hectares of area under organic farming, as per the FiBL (The Research Institute of Organic Agriculture) & IFOAM (International Federation of Organic Agriculture Movements) Organics International Report 2021. Madhya Pradesh has maximum land area under organic agriculture in the country and together with Rajasthan and Maharashtra account for about half the area under organic cultivation. India produced around 3430735.65

MT (2021-22) of certified organic products which includes all varieties of food products namely oil seeds, fibre, sugar cane, cereals & millets, cotton, pulses, aromatic & medicinal plants, tea, coffee, fruits, spices, dry fruits, vegetables, processed foods etc. The major exported organic food products were soya meal, oilseeds, cereals, millets sugar, tea & coffee spices and condiments, etc. The main importing countries of the country's organic produce were USA, European Union, Canada, Great Britain, Switzerland, Turkey, Australia, Ecuador, Korea Republic, Vietnam, Japan, etc. Organic food industry seems to be a promising future for Indian economics that has seen a major boost post-pandemic.

National Programme for Organic Farming

National Programme for Organic Production is an Indian Ministry of Commerce and Industry initiative, implemented in 2001. The programme involves the accreditation for certification bodies, standards for organic production, promotion of organic farming etc. The NPOP standards for production and accreditation system have been recognized by European Commission and Switzerland as equivalent to their country standards. Similarly, USDA has recognized NPOP conformity assessment procedures of accreditation as equivalent to that of US. The primary objectives of this programme are:

- Providing a platform or method that can evaluate the certification programme for organic agriculture and products, according to the criteria approved by the government.
- Recognizing the certification programmes of bodies that seek accreditation or certification.
- Facilitating the certification of organic products in compliance with approved standards.
- Helping the certification of organic products to be imported, as per the agreement of equivalence that is determined between the two nations, or in accordance with the requirement of the importing countries.
- Promoting organic farming, organic processing and their development in the country.

Standards Applicable for Organic Livestock Products

There is no single standard governing the organic foods globally at present; however it is restricted and may vary from country to country like UKROFS in UK, JAS in Japan, California organic standards in California, USA, AFRISCO standards in South Africa etc. There are following few international standards related to organic foods which are applicable all over the world:

1. IFOAM basic standards
2. EU regulations No. 1804/1999
3. Codex Alimentaruius ALINORM 99/22A

In India, Agricultural and Processed Food Products Export Development Authority (APEDA) under the *National Program for Organic Production* of the Government of India is responsible for certification and standards of organic livestock products produced and exported in India. Those standards ensures that the product or the raw materials used in the product were grown through organic farming, without the use of chemical fertilizers, pesticides, or induced hormones. Even though the standards are in effect since 2000, the certification scheme and hence the certification mark came into existence in 2002.

Certification System

The growing demand for organic produce has led to formulation of the certification systems for trusting quality of organic produce. Presently in India two types of certification system exists namely i.e. Third Party certification (NPOP) system and Participatory Guarantee System of India (PGS-INDIA) certification system. The Third Party certification is governed by APEDA, Ministry of Commerce which is mainly focused for export purpose and PGS-INDIA certification system is governed by Ministry of Agriculture and Farmers Welfare mainly deal with local/ domestic market. National Programme for Organic Production (NPOP) involves the accreditation of certification Bodies, standards for organic production, promotion of organic farming and marketing etc. The NPOP standards for production and accreditation system have been recognized by European Commission and Switzerland for unprocessed plant products as equivalent to their country standards. Presently there are 35 certified accredited bodies under NPOP. Products that meet NPOP standards can have – India Organics label printed on them. However, since India Organic is third party certification, besides India Organic logo it would also have *Name and logo of the Accredited Certification Body & Accreditation Number*. Under National Program for Organic Production System, a product can be labelled as Organic if:

- In case of single ingredient product where all requirements been met as per the specified standards can be labelled as 'Organic'.
- In case of multi ingredient product where min. 95% of ingredients are of certified origin, can be labelled as 'Certified Organic'

India Organic is a certification mark for organically farmed food products manufactured in India. The certification mark certifies that an organic food product confirms to the National Standards for Organic Products established in 2000.

PGS-INDIA was launched in 2011 by the Ministry of Agriculture and Farmers Welfare as an alternative to Third party (NPOP) certification system to make the certification system affordable and accessible without the need for third party certification agencies a farmer group centric certification system. PGS-India is a quality assurance initiative that is locally relevant, emphasizes the participation of stakeholders, including producers and consumers and operates outside the frame of third party certification. Both the programmes (NPOP and PGS-India) are independent of each other and products certified under one system cannot be processed or labeled under another system. NPOP certified products can be traded in export and in domestic market including imports, while PGS-India certified products can be traded only in domestic market.

FSSAI has also notified Food Safety and Standards (Organic Foods) Regulations, 2017 to ensure safety across the value chain through proper certification of organic foods.

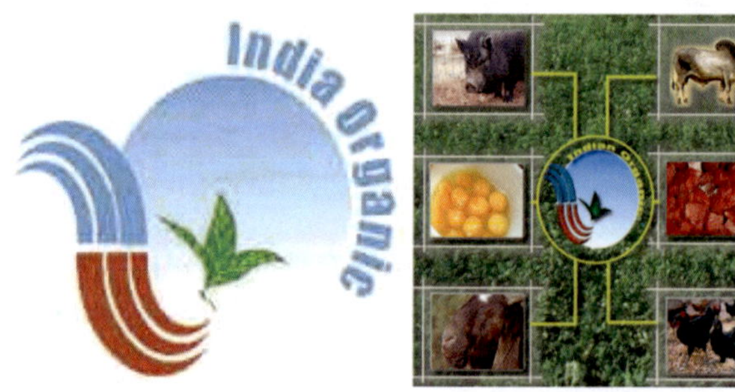

India Organic PGS-India Organic

Organic Goat Produce

Goat farming is a very profitable occupation for poor farmers as well as for that people who have a little or no other source of income including ladies. The main reason behind this the adapting nature of goat in various agro climatic conditions likearid dry to cold arid to hot humid. Goat farming requires low investment *i.e.* goats are small in size so need little space for rearing; they have got increased digestibility of crude fibre and can also survive in poor roughage ration (Boyazoglu et al., 2005). Goats are the multi-purpose animals in terms of production of meat, milk, hide, fibre and manure. There organic goat farming may be a useful strategy to achieve such a pivotal goal in terms of farms' profitability, environmental protection, food safety, and ethical concerns.Major considerations of organic goat production include personnel, livestock (animal welfare and health), facility, management, environmental conservation, product quality and safety, and profitability. Essential elements for a successful organic goat production may include nutrition and feeding, reproduction, breeding, animal health, animal welfare, environment, plants and vegetation and workers (Lu and Gangyi, 2008). Organic livestock products surged into the organic market place in the 1990s, establishing itself as a major category. In India it became visible much later and even till now there is no export of organic dairy and meat products at commercial level, therefore, it provides an immense opportunity for people involved in this industry to produce certified authentic organic livestock products.

Organic milk is the milk obtained from the animal that grazes on organic pastures for the entire season (at least 120 days in a year) and receives at least 30% of its nutrition from pastures. Animal must be fed high-forage diets with minimum forage content of 60-90%. Moroni et al. (2002)studied intramammary infections, milk productionand quality in organic dairy goat farming and concludedthat it is possible to control infections and somatic cellcounts without the use of drugs and maintain productionlevel and quality. The quantity of Organic milk obtained from organic farming is probably less due to lower energy intake and lower dry matter yields from organic pastures than the conventional farming. The quantity of fat in Organic milk may be more, less or same as that of conventional milk due to diet, breed of animal, stage of lactation, period of lactation, negative energy balance after calving, environment, seasonal variation (winter period), heritability, genotype etc. Rahmann (2008) studied the milking behavior of 20-35 lactating goats and reported a milk yield ranging from 488 to 790 kg/year, or 1.6 to 2.6 kg/day for a 305-day lactation period depending upon the pasture condition and fed intake. There is no obvious difference in production efficiency or carcass quality between organic and conventional goat herds. Zurita et al. (2008) studied 89 Murciano-Granadina kids from birth to 7 kg and reported a 0.5 kg difference between the conventional and organic herd. It is documented that Organic meat present a healthy profile for people of all ages since higher CLA and the lower ω-6:ω-3 ratio is beneficial characteristics for reducing the risk of chronic diseases, such as cardiovascular and other chronic inflammatory diseases. Organic meat cannot come into contact with nonorganic meat during processing and no synthetic materials can be used during the processing of organic meat and meat products. It is important to recognize that synthetic internal parasiticides on slaughter stock are not permitted. No synthetic materials including preservatives and flavoring agents can be used during the processing of organic milk and meat products. Information related to organic goat fiber and product processing is almost scarce.

Benefits of Organic Goat Farming

- Ensures strict animal welfare measures.
- Provides comfort to animal and favour the animal natural behaviour.
- Better for environmental safety and reduce pollution level.
- Better sustainability for production.
- Safe for consumption due to no use of Ab residues, pesticides, chemicals and drugs.
- Lower content of carcinogenic nitrogen and have potential to lower the incidences of cancer, coronary heart disease, allergies etc.
- Lower cost than conventional products.
- No use of genetically modified organisms, responsible for transgenic production.
- Fewer amounts of food additives and colouring agents in products. .
- Higher amount of nutrients.
- Challenges and Opportunities
- Sanitary regulations should be strictly monitored
- Prolong withdrawal period if any antibiotic or medicine is used.
- Delay in treatment of animals as treatment (naturopathy, Ayurveda and homeopathy).
- Processing and preservation of livestock produce is very difficult.
- Initial cost of production is very high.
- Infrastructure is not upto the mark and pure line herd is difficult to maintain.
- Very difficult to get rid of commonly occurring diseases.
- The procedure to get certification from agencies/ international bodies is complicated.
- Traceability is the biggest constraint for production of organic products.

Future Prospects

The demand for information is growing world over, for methods and practices of organic livestock farming. Goats are known as *"Wet nurse ofinfant"* in the United Kingdom and "Poor man`s cow"in India.Goat production is a dynamic andgrowing industry that is fundamental to thewellbeing of hundreds of millions of peopleworldwide. Consumers being more health-conscious, now prefer healthy, safe and nutritious foods with additional health promoting functions, such as organic livestock products. It has given an impetus to organic goat farming which can also be a good fit in developing countries. Global acceptance of organic products like goat cheeses, meat and fiber is also an important opportunity for the future growth of organic markets. While energy and chemical costs are high, practicing sustainable organic goat production in general has an economic edge. Alternative medicine as a result of prohibition of restricted materials to treat diseases and illness can be promising (Halberg et al., 2006). Epidemiological surveillance, emerging health issues, commercial traits for milk and meat production, biological control, animal welfare etc. have apparent research opportunities for production of organic goat produce. Organic goat farming provides opportunities for producers to match consumers′ preference in terms of wholesome and safe food, animal welfare, health and environmental protection at lower cost.

Conclusion

Organic livestock production is an emerging alternative to the intensive conventional livestock production systems, which is based on the development of harmonious relationship among soil, plants, animals and humans. Organic livestock production methods enhance the sustainability of agricultural production systems; produce healthy animals and quality livestock products while ensuring animal welfare and animal health. Organic goat farming may be a lucrative option for Indian farmers due to rich indigenous knowledge of livestock farming, rich biodiversity, availability of cheap labour, lower cost of production of organic dairy farming and with still unexplored vast domestic market conversion to organic production. Special attention must be paid on the production marketing strategies of organic products with linkage to government NGOs and corporate partnership.

References

BAHS (2022).https://dahd.nic.in/schemes/programmes/animal-husbandry-statistics

Bhattacharyya P. and Chakraborty G. (2005). Current status of organic farming in India and other countries. Indian Journal of Fertility.1 (9):111-123.

Boyazoglu, J., Hatziminaoglou, I. and Morand-Fehr, P. (2005). The role of the goat in society: Past, present and perspectives for the future. Small Ruminant Research. 60:13-23.

Chandan, R.C., Attaie, R. and Shahani, K.M. (1992). Nutritional aspects of goat milk and its products. Proceedings of 5th International Conference on Goats, March 2-8, New Delhi, India: 399-420.

Dhanda, J.S. (2001). Evaluation of crossbred goat genotypes for growth, carcass and meat quality characteristics. PhD Thesis, University of Queensland, Australia.

Haenlin, GFW. (1992). Role of goat meat and milk in human nutrition. Proceedings of 5th International Conference on Goats, March1-8, ICAR Publication: 575-580.

Halberg, N., Sulser, T.B., Høgh-Jensen, H., Rosegrant, M.W. and Knudsen, M.T. (2006). The impact of organic farming on food security in a regional and global perspective. In: Halberg, N., Alrøe, H.F., Knudsen, M.T., Kristensen, E.S. (Eds.), Global Development of Organic Agriculture: Challenges and Prospects. CABI Publishing, pp. 277–322

Hatziminaoglou, Y. and Boyazoglu, J. (2004). The goat in ancient civilizations: from the Fertile Crescent to the Aegean Sea. Small Ruminant Research. 51: 123–129

Kulhade, A., Gupta, A.D., Mishra, A. and Singh, S.R.K. (2016). Role of organic farming in Indian agriculture. 22(1):41-48.

Lu, C.D. and Gangyi, X. (2008). Organic sheep and goat production. In: Presented at Annual Meeting of Chinese Sheep and Goat Association, Zinben, Shannxi, China, July 22–25

Moroni, P., Bronzo, V., Cuccuru, C., Luzi, F., Cattaneo, D. and Savoini, G. (2002). Organic dairy goat farming: intramammary infections, milk production and quality. Organic meat and milk from ruminants. In: Proceedings of a Joint International Conference Organised by the Hellenic Society of Animal Production and the British Society of Animal Science, Athens, Greece, 4–6 October 2001.

Rahmann, G. (2008). Goat milk production under organic farming standards. In: Proceedings of the 9th International Conference on Goats,Queretaro, Mexico, August 31–September 4, p. 109.

Zurita, P., Camacho, M.E., Pleguezuelos, J. and Delgado, J.V. (2008). Organic vs. conventional herd effects on the weights and daily gains in Murciano- Granadina kids. In: Proceedings of the 9th International Conference onGoats, Queretaro, Mexico, August 31–September 4, p. 108.

10

Natural Goat Farming Practices in Uttrakhand: Opportunities and Challenges

J.P. Dhuliya

Dehradun, Uttarakhand

Natural goat farming is one among various farming systems that are close to nature and sustainability. In Uttrakhand which has 13-15 lakh goats as per animal husbandry department goat farming or rearing mimics how an animal would behave if they were freely living in the wild which therefore provides a more humane experience for the animal.In Uttrakhand, districts like Uttarkashi, Joshimath etc goat rearing is a part of indigenous lifestyle and tradition and is passed down generationally. They operate on no cost or low cost models therefore by default it is close to natural farming. They allow their goats to graze in forests and bugyal which are free from pesticides and fertilizers.Natural goat farming shall aim to use natural breeding methods, minimize stress, taking preventative measures and thereby eliminate the use of allopathic drugs or minimalist use of drug and detain animal health and welfare.Breed selection in natural goat farming should be indigenous as it is genetically adapted to specific or extreme conditions. They will be more productive and production cost will be lower.

Naturally raised goat meat is higher in protein and lower in fat. It also contains higher rates of omega-3 fatty acids and more antioxidants. Meanwhile, the taste of natural raised meat is delicious as per the customer reports.As we know in natural farming goats should behave like they would if they were freely grazing in the wild. Hence the concept of rotational grazing is introduced. Rotational grazing contributes to Pasture Health- Pasture has time to regenerate while goat manure acts as a natural fertilizer helping to restore vital nutrients for grass, legume and weeds growth.

- Animal Health- Constant access to fresh pasture means that the goats are grazing on a wide variety of their natural food source.

- Human Health- Healthier animals produce healthier meat.
- Environmental Health- Goats graze plants that have absorbed Co2 from the air but due to rotational grazing the goats move to fresh pasture ensuring that no one section of land is overgrazed, allowing the land to rest in between grazing cycles and regenerate.

Natural Goat Farming Management

- Goats have to be in fresh air, daylight and have some freedom to roam inside or outside.
- Dry bedding or raised wooden pellets must be there.
- Availability of good forages in outdoor areas strengthens the natural immune system.
- Availability of fresh water.
- Excellent vaccination program and record keeping.
- No caging and tethering.
- No overcrowding.
- Emphasis on preventative measures and strengthening immune systems.
- Using alternative medicines like ayurveda and homeopathy.
- Conventional veterinary medicine should be used in case of emergency. If used, thewithholding period of milk or meat should be twice the legal, essential period.

Opportunities

Increasing income, changing diets and population growth have led to increased demand and made the livestock sector one of the fastest growing. The demand for organic/natural raised meat products will increase in the future as health awareness especially after COVID-19 has increased. We have to convey the benefits of natural/organic raised meat through print media, social media and dedicated government organizations. By doing this we can develop our domestic market and later on may target USA and European countries which constitute 95% of the organic market.

Challenges

- Per day weight gain is less as compared to grain fed thus the time period for farmers to sell their products will be more.
- During the dry season (Mid February to June) the goats feed on low qualitygrasses/shrubs and have low protein diets hence low weight gain.

- Establishing protocols and promoting natural livestock production and its certification in India
- Invasion of *Lantana Camara* in forests. Due to this forests and grasslands are shrinking. It does not allow any vegetation to grow around it.
- In their natural habitat, goats are always prone to predators.
- As forests and grasslands are limited, practicing additional grazing becomesproblematic.

11

Natural Resource Based Feeding for Goats

Ravindra Kumar*, Mohd. Arif and Shilpi Gupta

Principal Scientist (Animal Nutrition), Division of Animal Nutrition Management and PT ICAR-CIRG, Makhdoom, Farah, Mathura Uttar Pradesh

Goat (*Capra hircus*) is a domesticated species of goat-antelope typically kept as livestock. It was domesticated from the wild goat (*C. aegagrus*) of Southwest Asia and Eastern Europe. It is one of the oldest domesticated species of animal, according to archaeological evidence that its earliest domestication occurred in Iran at 10,000 calibrated calendar years ago. Beginning approximately 10,000 years ago, Neolithic farmers in the Near East started keeping small herds of goats for both their meat and milk, as well as for clothing and building with the hair, bone, skin and power. Undoubtedly, goat farming at the time was natural resource based and is organic in nature. Mechanical (1880–1930) and chemical (1920–1950) revolutions in agriculture, significantly influenced the modern day livestock farming predominately in non-organic form. Biological advances in the genetically modified organisms in the 70s further complicated the researcher–producer–consumer dynamics. As of today, there are over 750 million goats scattered throughout the world. Goats are found in nearly every country on the planet and in nearly every climate, each one with a different purpose. There are more than a thousand adapted breeds in existence. Goats have been used for milk, meat, fur, and skins across much of the world.

Feeding behaviour of goats

Goats are efficient browsers and prefer eating brushy plants along with some other woody and weedy plants found on the ranges. Goats are able to digest a large variety of fibre and roughage. The nutrient requirements of goats are determined by age, sex, breed, production system (dairy or meat), body size, climate and physiological stage. Feeding strategies should be able to meet energy, protein, mineral, and vitamin needs depending on the condition of the goats. Goats do not depend on intensive feeding systems except some supplemental feeding during growth, lactation, pregnancy and winter. Of course, when goats are in lactation for an extended period of time (around 10 months), they will require supplemental feeding on a higher plane of nutrition. Goats belong to the small ruminant group of animals and have no upper incisor or canine teeth but a dental pad instead. The rumen is the largest part of four stomach compartments with the capacity of roughly 2-6 pounds. Some bacteria and protozoa are normal habitants of the rumen which break down plant food into volatile fatty acids along with vitamins and amino acids. The daily feed intake of goat's ranges from 3-4% of body weight as expressed in pounds (dry matter/head/day). The daily feed intake is influenced by body weight, % of dry matter in the feeds eaten (12-35% in forages, 86-92% in hays and concentrate's), palatability, and physiological stage of the goats (growth, pregnancy, and lactation).

Goats are ruminant's animals with a four compartment stomach. The 4 parts in a goat's stomach are the reticulum, rumen, omasum and abomasum, or the "true stomach When they eat, food first goes through microbial digestion in the reticulum and rumen. Then, it goes through an acidic breakdown in the abomasum. Finally, it undergoes enzymatic digestion and absorption in the intestines. Interestingly, when a goat is first born, it has 3 stomach compartments. This is so they can absorb the antibodies in colostrum and develop the microbes and bacteria needed for digestion. They then develop the 4th part when they start eating high-fiber foods. There are a lot of benefits to a ruminant's complex digestive system. The microbial digestion makes it possible for them to eat a high-fiber diet and digest grass, hay, leaves, etc. They can also eat bark, weeds and woody plants that cattle and sheep can't. This is because the bacteria in their rumen detoxify anything that isn't nutritious and even helps to detoxify some poisons. The bacteria also utilize and absorb all of the B vitamins that they need, which is something that's hard to do, even for humans. The bacteria in their stomachs convert nitrogen into protein, which is a handy feature to have considering they don't naturally eat much protein on their own.

Feeding Resources

Among all the ruminants, goats are only the animals which can eat and consume almost all types of food. Goat can be raised by providing all types of natural, home or commercially formulated goat feed. Nowadays goat farming is becoming very popular because of its multifunctional utility. But the profitable production from goat farming business mostly depends on proper feed supply and management systems. Proper feed management includes providing nutritious food, vitamins, minerals, energy, protein etc.

Pasture

In Indian condition majority of goats derive their nutrients from pasture browsing. By browsing pasture, goats will remain healthy and will get sufficient and necessary food elements like energy and protein. Natural food from pasture also helps the goats increasing the tastiness and digestibility of other foods. A pasture with natural plants and grasses like millet, Sudan grasses, Bahia grasses, grain grass mixture, clover, sorghum etc. are very healthy and effective for goat's production and health. In pasture if the goats can browse freely then it will help them to keep free from various internal and external parasitical diseases. Strategic supplementation of tree leaves to pasture goats can improve the productivity and reduce the methane production also. In our lab we have found that Methane emission (g/day) was significantly ($P<0.05$) reduced on Subabul (*Leucenea leucocephala*) supplementation in grazing goats. *In vivo* methane emission (g/day) decreased by 18.30 % on subabool supplementation. Reduction in the methane production may be due to improvement in nutrient utilization and rumen fermentation on supplementation of Subabul which is a source of plant secondary metabolites like tannins and other nutrients. These tree leaves are a source of plant secondary metabolites which have a methane suppressing effect in ruminants.

Hay

Hay is another important source of goat nutrition, especially in winter seasons. There are various types of hays are available. Among those lespedeza, alfalfa and clover hays are highly enriched in protein and some other essential nutrients.

Moringa

Moringa *(Moringa oleifera)* is a rapidly growing soft wood plant that is mainly distributed in tropical and subtropical zones. India is the largest producer of Moringa and a yield up to 650 metric tonnes of green leaves per hectare can be achieved using optimum conditions for the cultivation (Rajangam *et al.*, 2001). *Moringa oleifera* leaves are rich source of protein (23-30%), minerals, vitamins and other secondary metabolites (Su and Chen, 2020). Fresh *M. oleifera* leaves at 20 and 50% levels as a replacement for batiki grass (*Ischaemum aristatum* var. *indicum*) improved live weight gain and nutrient digestibility in growing goats (Aregheore, 2002). Moringa (*M. olifera*) is highly nutritious & economic fodder for goat due to its high biomass production. Moringa (*Moringa oleifera*) can be grown as perennial multi-cut fodder crop and it can produce good quality green fodder. ICAR-CIRG, Makhdoom is growing moringa as a fodder crops in nearly 10 acres of area for goats and sheep. Once it established it provides green fodder up 3-4 years. In moringa, the first cut is taken 90 days after sowing and subsequent cuts at 60 days interval. While cutting, it is desirable to leave a height of at least 20-30 cm from the ground level so as to avoid damage to the young growing roots near the base of the plant. The growth of the plant is checked in winter months when the cold is very severe, but starts sprouting again as soon as it warms up. Kumar *et al*. (2023) evaluated green moringa (*Moringa olifera*) foliage in growing Barbari goats under stall feeding. Growing female Barbari goats were fed *ad libitum* green moringa and supplemented concentrate pellet (1.5% of body weight). The average daily dry matter intake was 490.86 g comprising of 234.83 g green moringa and 256.03 g concentrate pellet. The average daily gain of female goats was 54.26 g. The feed conversion ratio was 9.94. The average calculated cost per kg weight gain was Rs. 125.50. Blood metabolites viz., glucose, total protein, albumin, globulin, serum enzymes (*aspartate aminotransferase*, alanine aminotransferase) and ruminal volatile fatty acids were within normal range. *Ad lib* green moringa feeding along with supplemental concentrate pellet was found economic option for feeding of growing goats at our institute.

Tripathi *et al*. (2014) reported that *Tephrosia purpurea, Cenchrus ciliaris* and *Dactylotennium aegypticum* monsoon herbages had the potential of feeding during post monsoon season to kids for optimum growth. The *Tephrosia purpurea* being the leguminous forage had higher CP and better nutrients density, while *Cenchrus ciliaris* and *Dactylotennium aegypticum* had the higher palatability to cater the need for optimum growth.

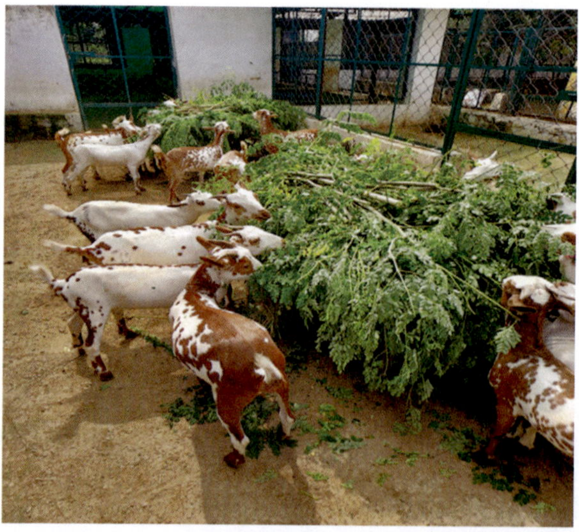

Azolla

Azolla a free-floating aquatic fern which fixes atmospheric nitrogen in association with nitrogen fixing blue green alga *Anabaena azollae*, making it an excellent source of protein for livestock. It belongs to the family *Azollaceae* and order Pteridophyta. The plant is highly productive with the ability to double its weight in seven days. It can produce 9 tonnes of protein per hectare of pond per year. This can be used as a part of feed or as a supplemental source of protein and minerals in the ration of goats. Azolla in the complete feed can reduce the cost of feed of goat there by increasing the profits from goat rearing to the farmers. Azolla was found to contain 78-80 % organic matter, 17-22 % crude protein, 2-3 % crude fat and 12-15% crude fibre on dry matter basis. The per cent NDF and ADF of azolla recorded was 45-47 and 30-33 respectively. Sodium, potassium, calcium (%) was 0.60, 0.73, 0.11 while Copper and zinc (ppm) was 16.12 and 71.47 respectively indicating azolla as a good source of macro as well as micro minerals (Kumar *et al.*, 2015). Fresh azolla can be fed to growing and adult goats. Fresh azolla harvested can be mixed with straw and fed to the goats. The rate of incorporation of azolla should be 50-100 gm/day in growing animals and 100-200 gm/day in the adult animals. Azolla can be harvested and sundried for storage and feeding to goats. Sundried azolla can be mixed in the concentrate mixture as a replacement of concentrate mixture in the goat ration. This will economize the feeding cost of goats because the ingredient cost of concentrate mixture is quite high. Supplementation of Azolla has been found o improve the milk production in goats without any significant effect on milk composition (Kumar *et al.*, 2022).

Tree Foliage and Fallen Leaves Feeding

The shortage of feed during the long dry season in tropics and subtropics is one of the major constraints in maintaining/ enhancing productivity of ruminant livestock. Crop residues, such as straw, that constitutes the bulk of the feed supply in tropical animal farming systems are characterized by a high percentage of cell wall components, low quantities of protein and minerals. Low total digestibility, slow rate of breakdown of straw particles to a size that can leave the rumen, low propionate fermentation pattern in the rumen and the negligible content of both fermentable N and by-pass protein are major associated limitations with straws. A feed containing less than 6% crude protein promotes negative N balance owing to protein malnutrition and therefore, require N supplementation to improve microbial protein synthesis in rumen. During draught, even these poor feed resources remain in short supply. Tree leaves, which are rich in nitrogen and widely used in the tropics, offer the opportunity for use as N supplements to livestock fed on crop residues. Fallen tree leaves (FTL) are often responsible for forest fire. However, this resource might be used as source of roughage especially during summer season (feed scarcity period) or during draught. Inclusion of fallen tree leaves up to 20% in complete feed block without any adverse effect on intake, digestibility, rumen fermentation pattern and general health of the animals has been reported. Further, it is also observed that tree, shrubs and bushes are highly preferred by goats. In case of tree fodder tannin is one of the limiting factors in leaves. However, lopping of the fodder trees can be used as a source of fodder if it is used up to level *i.e.* up to 30% of total dry matter intake (Dutta, 2009).

Table 1: Fodder availability periods in important fodder tress

Tree species	Fodder availability period		Preference to livestock
	Leaf Fodder	Pod fodder	
Acacia nilotica	May - February	April - June	Cattle, Goat, Sheep, camel
Ailanthus excelsa	May - March	-	Goat, Sheep
Albizia lebbek	April - November	August- November	Goat, Sheep, Cattle
Azadirachta indica	Though out the year	July – August	Goat, Sheep, Cattle
Bauhinia variegata	April- November	-	Goat, Sheep, Cattle
Dalbergia sissoo	February-December	April- September	Goat, Sheep, Cattle
Ficus religiosa	July - November		Sheep, Cattle
Hardwickia binata	April- June	February- March	Cattle, Sheep, Goat
Leucaena leucocephala	Throughout the year	December- May	Cattle, Goat, Sheep
Melia azedarach	July - November	-	Goat, Sheep, Cattle
Prosopis cineraria	Throughout the year	May- June	Goat, Sheep, Camel Cattle
Sesbania grandiflora	July- November	-	Cattle, Sheep, Goat
Sesbania sesban	Throughout the year	December- March	Cattle, Goat, Sheep
Ziziphus mumularia	Throughout the year	-	Cattle, Goat, Sheep

(*Source*: Rai *et al.*, 2007)

The most common fodder tree species for small ruminants are khejri, siris, ardu, babul, bakain, pakar, gular, pipal, bargad, sesbania, subabul, neem, shahtut, kharjal, kathal etc. *Khejri*leaves aresmall in size but highly nutritive and palatable. Theses leaves locally known as "Loong" and it is very much liked by goats. The leaves of *Siris* tree are also reported to be good for goat rearing purposes. *Ardu* leaves are excellent tree fodder with high palatability and nutritious for sheep and goat (Mann and Sharma, 2006). *Babul*leaves are also excellent fodder and extensively lopped for fodder. *Bakain*leaf fodder is highly nutritious and can be used for supplementing the sheep and goat ration. The leaves of *Pakar* are highly nutritious and palatable. The total digestible nutrients are more in young leaves. *Gular*is also extensively lopped for fodder. *Pipal* leaves rated as a good fodder. Goat relishes the leaves and palatability of the leaves for other animals is also fairly good. *Bargad* leaves are very much liked by goats as compared to other animals. *Sesbania grandiflora* leaves and pods can be used as a valuable fodder for ruminants. Due to high protein content, it can be combined with poor quality roughages and intake can be increased by supplementing it. *Subabul* leaves are the good source of carotene and vitamins. Subabul leaf meal is specially valuable due to its amino acid content which is superior to other plant proteins and it is almost as good as lucerne (Tripathi *et al.*, 2009). *Neem* leaves provide enough nutrients and can very well use as a green fodder supplement (Mann and Sharma, 2006). *Shahtut* leaves are good fodder and can profitably utilize as a supplement to poor quality roughages. These leaves are highly palatable to sheep. *Kharjal/ Pilu* leaves and young shoots are browsed by the goats and sheep. *Kathal* leaves are very well consumed by sheep and goat.

Organic Goat Production

Main thoughts of organic goat production include personnel, livestock (animal welfare and health), facility, management, environmental conservation, product quality and safety, and profitability. Essential elements for a successful organic goat production may include nutrition and feeding, reproduction, breeding, animal health, animal Welfare, environment, plants and vegetation and workers (Lu and Gangyi, 2008).

In summary, pastures must be certified organic and maintained without the use of pesticides, herbicides, chemical fertilizers, or other restricted materials. Anything fed (hay, grain, pellets, and milk replacer) to does and kids must be certified organic. Organically grown feed cannot contain synthetic hormones, antibiotics, coccidiostats, urea, or other restricted materials. Even bedding, which may be consumed by animals, must be certified organic.

Animals intended for slaughter cannot be treated with antibiotics, anthelmintic, growth implants, or other prohibited materials. Breeding stock can be dewormed only with Ivermectin on the basis of fecal egg counts, but not on a routine or preventative basis and not during lactation. Animals which must be treated with prohibited materials cannot be represented as organic. Vaccinations are acceptable. Records must be maintained on feed and health care. Identification of animals is required throughout the life cycle. Organically-produced animal is not the same as naturally-raised, free-range, or grass-fed (Lu and Gangyi, 2008).

The majority of the goats kept in villages are seldom given any grain or good fodder, as a result their average milk production is very low. Milch goats respond readily to good care and proper feeding, and to ensure best results they should be tended like other milch animals. The availability, quality, and cost of feeds have been identified as the major constraints to acceptable livestock productivity across the various regions. Nutrition is the most limiting factor for goats in India to accomplish their genetic potential. Most Indian goats are managed in extensive grazing systems and information about goat nutrition and management practices in India is limited.

Milk Production

It has been established that organic dairy goat production can be productive and sustainable. Rahmann (2002) described an annual average milk yield from 532 to 835 g/day of a herd with 20–35 lactating goats over a period of 6 years in Germany. Though, the availability of forage, affected by rainfall and other environmental factors, contributed to the fluctuation in milk yield over a 6-year period. In a more recent study/survey with a larger herd over a 4-year period, Rahmann (2008) reported a milk yield ranging from 488 to 790 kg/year, or 1.6 to 2.6 kg/day for a 305-day lactation period. These reports established that higher yields are possible in organic dairy goat production, but is subject to pasture condition. In much of the developing world, goat milk is the primary milk source for humans. Goat milk is often sought for its perceived health benefits and unique taste. Although many health effects have been attributed to consuming goat milk, scientific evidence does not support most health claims. Goat milk is similar in composition to cow milk, but some important differences exist in the protein structure. Because of these differences, people who have allergies to cow milk can often drink goat milk, and the smaller fat globules in goat milk stay in suspension longer, which leads to the perception of "natural homogenization." Goats are excellent browsers, which allows them to consume plants containing aromatic or flavour compounds that can impart the smell or flavour to the milk or cheese, thus providing an opportunity to generate unique specialty products.

During processing, organic milk is not allowed to be contaminated by chemicals. No synthetic materials that include preservatives and flavouring agents can be used during the processing of organic milk and other dairy products. It is legal to use raw milk in making cheese if the cheese is aged at least 60 days before sale (Dairy Practices Council, 1994). Fresh cheese must be made with pasteurized milk.

Meat Production

Goats are prolific and resilient small ruminant livestock with a wide ecological adaptation. Production and consumption of goat meat are low despite the importance of the species, but this sector has huge potential to supply food for a growing human population. Goat meat serves as a major source of meat in developing countries while it is less popular in western countries. Nevertheless, the perceptions about goat meat are changing due to the health benefits of the consumption of lean meat with reduced fat and cholesterol content.

There is no obvious difference in production efficiency or carcass quality between organic and conventional goat herds. Guzman et al. (2008) used 24 identical twins and studied the carcass yield in Blanca Andaluza kids from birth to 8.4 kg. They reported differences in leg compactness index, offal distribution, but no difference in carcass yield and conformation. Zurita et al. (2008) studied 89 Murciano Granadina kids from birth to 7 kg and reported a 0.5 kg difference between the conventional and organic herd. Organic goat meat production generally favours a feeding system that avoids a high energy diet with maximum weight gain. As a result, the carcass will likely accumulate less amount of internal fat around their heart and kidneys. A slower rate of gain, but heavier market weight, is therefore more advisable.

Organic meat cannot come into contact with nonorganic meat during processing and no synthetic materials can be used during the processing of organic meat and meat products. It is important to recognize that synthetic internal parasiticides on slaughter stock are not permitted. Instead, a program based on fecal exams, culling of seriously infested animals, pasture rotation, manure management and vector and intermediate host control using allowed materials should be considered.

Nutritional Implications in Organic Goat

Nutritional implications in parasitic control in goats have been studied (Hoste et al., 2005). It has been verified that protein supplementation can improve resistance or resilience of grazing goats. This is important, as the control of parasites and other diseases can be a challenge in organic goat production. A boost in the immune system as a result of protein supplementation can develop the production efficiency of organic goat herds. Since of the importance in synchronization of energy and protein to achieve optimal microbial synthesis in the rumen, an optimum energy and protein interaction is important in organic goat production (Lu and Potchoiba, 1990). This can be challenging when goats are on pasture and rely mainly on grazing. Understanding of nutrition, eating behaviour and seasonal interaction can also be beneficial to improve production efficiency (Lu, 1988; Torres-Acosta et al., 2000).

Secondary metabolites such as tannins and tanniferous plants have implications in organic goat production. Trichostrongyle egg excretion in naturally infected goats was significantly less when sainfoin was included in the diet . Tannin reduced fecal egg counts in goats. Lespedeza with high condensed tannins reduced fecal egg count and mortality rate in meat goats. Effects of dehydrated neem, fresh neem, and seed extracts on fecal egg counts were inconclusive (Luginbuhl and Pietrosemoli, 2008). Heather supplementation reduced fecal egg counts in goats (Osoro et al., 2007). The authors suggested that heather availability in the vegetation might represent a valuable opportunity and sustainable method to control gastrointestinal nematode infections in a goat production systems based on grazing perennial ryegrass-white clover pastures. The effect of natural zeolite that reduced fecal egg counts had been recently reviewed (Papaioannou et al., 2005).Legumes can be important in organic goat farming systems. It is attributed to their abilities in nitrogen fixation, increased soil fertility and stability, capacity for nutrient recycling, control of weed species, break disease and pest life cycles, high protein animal feed cash crop, biodiversity and landscape quality, and operational flexibility (Howieson et al., 2000).

Grazing management strategies are also important in the control of internal parasites and diseases. These include preventive (turning out parasite free animals on clean pastures), evasive (worm challenge is evaded by moving animals from contaminated to clean pastures) and diluting (worm challenge is relieved by diluting pasture infectivity) strategies.

Conclusion

Natural goat production systems are more sustainable with more animal welfare, protect to environment, and reward a higher product price to the goat owner. Feed and nutrition being an important component of production system should also be taken into account. Natural feed resources can provide the nutrients along with some health promoting effect to the goats.

References

Aregheore, E.M. 2002. Intake and digestibility of Moringa oleifera–batiki grass mixtures by growing goats. Small Ruminant Research, 46:23–8. doi: 10.1016/S0921-4488(02)00178-5.

Dairy Practices Council, 1994. Guidelines for Production and Regulation of Quality Dairy Goat Milk. DPC Publication No. 59, p. 17.

Dutta, T. K. 2009. Nutritional management of goats for commercial production. In Goat Enterprises edited by Shalander Kumar, M.C. Sharma and A.K. Goel. 2009.Published by Published by Central institute for Research on Goats, Makhdoom, Mathura -281122 (Uttar Pradesh), India pp: 90-106.

Guzmán, J.L., Delgado-Pertínez, M., Zarazaga, L.A., Flores, A., Puerta, R., Celi, I., Acosta, J.M., Argüello, A., 2008. Effect of management system on the regional composition and offal distribution in Blanca Andaluza goat kids. In: Proceedings of the 9th International Conference on Goats, Queretaro, Mexico, August 31–September 4, pp. 113–114.

Hoste, H., Torres-Acosta, J.F., Paolini, V., Aguilar-Caballero, A., Etter, E., Lefrileux, Y., Chartier, C., Broqua, C., 2005. Interactions between nutrition and gastrointestinal infections with parasitic nematodes in goats. Small Rumin. Res. 60, 141–151

Howieson, J.G., O'Hara, G.W., Carr, S.J., 2000. Changing roles for legumes in Mediterranean agriculture: developments from an Australian perspective. Field Crops Res. 65, 107–122.

Kumar Ravindra, Abraham, G., Jaiswal, P. and Verma, A.K. 2022. Effect of green Azolla supplementation on milk production, constituents and fatty acids profile in mid-lactating Barbari goats. Indian Journal of Dairy Science, 75: 478-481.

Kumar Ravindra, Dixit, A.K., Kumar, A. and Sharma, D.K. 2023. Nutritional evaluation of Green Moringa (Moringa olifera) foliage in Barbari goats. Indian journal of small ruminants, 29: 152-154.

Kumar Ravindra, Tripathi, P., Chaudhary, U.B. and Tripathi M.K. 2015. Nutrient composition, in vitro methane production and digestibility of Azolla (Azolla microphylla) with rumen liquor of goat. The Indian journal of small ruminants, 21: 126-128.

Lu, C.D., 1988. Grazing behaviour and diet selection of goats. Small Rumin. Res. 1, 205–216.

Lu, C.D., Gangyi, X., 2008. Organic sheep and goat production. In: Presented at Annual Meeting of Chinese Sheep and Goat Association, Zinben, Shannxi, China, July 22–25 (Invited Paper).

Lu, C.D., Potchoiba, M.J., 1990. Feed intake and weight gain of growing goats feed diets of various energy and protein levels. J. Anim. Sci. 68, 1751–1759.

Luginbuhl, J.-M., Pietrosemoli, S., 2008. Use of dehydrated neem (Azadirachta indica A. Juss) leaves to control coccidiosis in young goats. In: Proceedings of the 9th International Conference on Goats, Queretaro, Mexico, August 31–September 4, p. 270.

Mann, J.S. and Sharma, S. C. 2006. Lean period forages in arid and semi-arid zones of India. In : Livestock feeding strategies for dry regions. Editors P S Pathak and S S Kundu, ISBN no. 81-8189-127-9 pp: 399- 428.

Osoro, K., Mateos-Sanz, A., Frutos, P., García, U., Ortega-Mora, L.M., Ferreira, L.M.M., Celaya, R., Ferre, I., 2007. Anthelmintic and nutritional effects of heather supplementation on Cashmere goats grazing perennial ryegrass-white clover pastures. J. Anim. Sci. 85, 861–870.

Papaioannou, D., Katsoulos, P.D., Panousis, N., Karatzias, H., 2005. The role of natural and synthetic zeolites as feed additives on the prevention and/or the treatment of certain farm animal diseases: a review. Micropor. Mesopor. Mater. 84, 161–170.

Rahmann, G., 2002. On farm organic dairy sheep and goat breeding in Germany. In: Proceedings of the 14th IFOAM Organic World Congress, p. 94.

Rahmann, G., 2008. Goat milk production under organic farming standards. In: Proceedings of the 9th International Conference on Goats, Queretaro, Mexico, August 31–September 4, p. 109

Rai, P., Ajit and Samanta, A. K. 2007. Tree leaves, their production, and nutritive value for ruminants: A review. Animal Nutrition and Feed Technology, 7: 135-139.

Rajangam, J., Azhakiamanavalan, R. S., Thangaraj, T., Vijayakumar ,A. and Muthukrishnan, N. 2001. Status of production and utilisation of moringa in Southern India. Proceedings of the Development potential for moringa products held at Tanzania, March 2001.

Su, B. and Chen, X.2020. Current status and potential of Moringa oleifera leaf as an alternative protein source for animal feeds. Frontiers in Veterinary Science, 7:1-13.

Torres-Acosta, J.F.J., Jacobs, D.E., Aguilar-Caballero, A.J., 2000. Effect of supplementary feeding on the resilience of Criollo kids browsing under tropical condition. Round Table 6. Integrated control of nematode parasites. In: Proceedings of the Seventh International Conference on Goats, 14–20 May 2000, Tours, France, p. 807.

Tripathi, P. Dutta, T. K., Chaudhary, U. B. and Sharma, M. C. 2009. Tree leaves for small ruminant production in semi-arid and arid zones of North India. Published by Central institute for Research on Goats, Makhdoom, Mathura -281122 (Uttar Pradesh), India.

Tripathi Prabhat ,Dutta T.K., Tripathi M.K., Chaudhary U.B., Kumar Ravindra, 2014. Preparartion of complete feed pellet from monsoon herbages. D. aegypticum, C. ciliaris and T. Purpurea and its utilization in kids. Indian journal of Small ruminants, 20: 31-36.

Zurita, P., Camacho, M.E., Pleguezuelos, J., Delgado, J.V., 2008. Organic vs. conventional herd effects on the weights and daily gains in MurcianoGranadina kids. In: Proceedings of the 9th International Conference on Goats, Queretaro, Mexico, August 31–September 4, p. 108.

12

Role of ICT and Extension Services in three Phase Goat Production System

R.P. Dwivedi, Priyanka Singh, Asharam, A.K. Handa Sushil Kumar and A. Arunachalam

ICAR- Central Agroforestry Research Institute, Jhansi, Uttar Pradesh

Goat is considered as KAMDHENU of small and marginal farmers in India. Agroforestry plays a very important role in three phase goat production system for the demand for natural/organic livestock product. Three phase goat production system i.e. extensive system, semi-intensive system and intensive system are very much supported by agroforestry systems. Goat farming contributes significantly to the family economy, sustainable livelihoods and poverty.

Agroforestry is a collective name for land-use systems and technologies where woody perennials (trees, shrubs, palms, bamboos, etc.) are deliberately used on the same land-management units as agricultural crops and/or animals, in some form of spatial arrangement or temporal sequence. In agroforestry systems there are both ecological and economical interactions between the different components. Agroforestry can also be defined as a dynamic, ecologically based, natural resource management system that, through the integration of trees on farms and in the agricultural landscape, diversifies and sustains production for increased social, economic and environmental benefits for land users at all levels. In particular, agroforestry is crucial to smallholder farmers and other rural people because it can enhance their food supply, income and health. Agroforestry systems are multifunctional systems that can provide a wide range of economic, sociocultural, and environmental benefits. (FAO, 2015)

Agroforestry has been defined in several ways (Nair, 1989). ICRAF's current definition is a collective name for land-use systems and practices in which woody perennials are deliberately integrated with crops and/or animals on the same land-management unit.

In simple words, Agroforestry is equal to Tree plus Crop plus Livestock together practiced at farmers' field for better economic returns, livelihood options and ecosystem restoration.

Tree + Crop + Livestock = Agroforestry (Dwivedi, 2015).

Lakdi Chara Phal Aur Ann - Krishivaniki hai Jeevan

Agroforestry has always been an integral part of the Indian culture owing to the long standing social, ethnic and religious significance of trees in the country. Several forms of traditional agroforestry practices are prevalent in different parts of India; however recognition of trees as an important component of farming systems remains limited. India became the first country in the world to adopt National Agroforestry Policy on 10th Feb, 2014 and has a well organized institutional framework for promoting agroforestry research and education activities. At the national level, Central Agroforestry Research Institute (CAFRI) functioning under Indian Council of Agricultural Research play a proactive role in agroforestry research and education activities. The Indian Council of Forestry Research and Education (ICFRE) that was set up along the lines of ICAR has also contributed to agroforestry research in the past years. At the state level, the state agricultural, horticultural, forestry, veterinary and animal sciences universities have also catered the agroforestry research needs in a substantial manner. Besides these public functionaries, several private and non-governmental organizations are also involved in research and outreach activities that are of relevance to agroforestry. However several bottlenecks exist in mainstreaming agroforestry for an *Atmanirbhar Bharat.* This paper articulates ways in which extension strategies can facilitate the successful adoption of modern and scientific agroforestry practices. The farmers should not be imposed any woody perennials and the farmer's preference should be taken into consideration before recommending tree species (Dwivedi, et al 2007). The location of tree plantation is also important in promotion of agroforestry. The field/farm boundary system of agroforestry has been widely practiced in traditional as well as commercial agroforestry regions (Dwivedi, et al 2013). Agroforestry is also playing an important role in fulfilling the SDGs of the United Nations and one of the top solutions for climate change.

One of the basic objectives of National Agroforestry Policy – 2014 (India) is to encourage and expand the tree plantation in complementarity and integrated manner with crops and livestock to improve productivity, employment, income and livelihoods of rural households, especially the small farmers. ICAR-CAFRI's vision 2050 says that major role for agroforestry in near future will be in the domain of environmental services and watershed protection.

In India, we do not have much more land to expand the forest and on the other side as per National Forest Policy 1988, we have to have one-third of the country's geographical area under forest and tree cover for maintaining ecological balance and environmental equilibrium. The big question is how to solve the problem? The ANSWER lies in Agroforestry. In this direction, National Agroforestry Policy -2014 is a ray of hope to have one-third tree cover outside the forest area by promotion and adoption of agroforestry.

Extension Education Strategy

Extension Education Strategy is a plan that you use in order to achieve dissemination of awareness and creating interest for adoption of agroforestry technologies at farmers' fields. The Vision of the Agroforestry Extension Strategy is to ensure conditions for the dissemination and exchange of information between farmers, producers, agroforestry experts and other stakeholders in order to transform the agroforestry so that this can contribute effectively to economic returns, livelihood options and ecosystem restoration.

The following ICT and extension services will be applicable to motivate farmers to adopt goat production based agroforestry on farmers' field:

1. **Organizing short courses to develop a cadre of agroforestry ambassadors:** Besides organizing field days and agroforestry expo, the institute can plan short duration courses that are directly relevant to the farm and that aim at building the competencies of rural youth. Short modularized courses meeting specific needs for knowledge, skill and competencies should be developed with the main aim to impart experiential learning to farmers. For instance, in Australia University of Melbourne initiated a Master Tree Grower Programme (MTG) in which interested farmers are given a field based training for 8 days. Similarly ICAR-CAFRI can facilitate such short duration programmes, imparting knowledge on region specific successful agroforestry models, their package of practice, value addition and marketing. These farmers can in turn act as master trainers and give training to other farmers in their region, facilitating one to one information exchange and support linear technology transfer.
2. **Use of mass media (Print & Electronic) to create awareness among farmers and other stakeholders:** A critical review suggest that poorly targeted information, information overload and promulgation of unreliable information pose major challenge for the potential agroforestry stakeholders. Ready reckoners on successful agroforestry models and its economic, environment and social impact in different agroclimatic

zones must be made available in regional languages to create awareness and interest in the farmers. Developing a handbook of agroforestry, a comprehensive source that offers state-of-the-art knowledge of different aspects of agroforestry, advanced research results and evaluations, socio-economic and environmental aspects of agroforestry will be useful for the academicians, scientific faculty, students and other working professionals in the field of agroforestry. There should be regular TV show about agroforestry on DD Kisan.

3. **Developing expert system (Farm TreeApp) for promising tree species in the country:** Efforts can be made in this direction to address ad hoc information requirements of farmers. Expert system integrating precise and up-to-date information on tree choice, irrigation management, fertilizer recommendation, disease and pest diagnosis and market prices must be made available in local languages to assist the farmers in making informed decisions. Considering the limited number of agroforestry subject matter specialists in KVKs, development of expert system will help reach larger audience within less time, thus increasing the visibility and relevance of the public extension system.
4. **Agroforestry farmer field schools (AFFS) for capacity building of farmers:** Farmer field schools is a widely accepted concept due to its participatory nature. A key principle of AFFS is transferring knowledge produced from research institutes to the farmers through active participation of research institutes, extension workers and farmers in the entire process.
5. **Felicitating progressive Goat farmers:** Innovative and progressive Goat farmers can be invited and felicitated on days like Agroforestry Day, World Forestry Day, World Environment Day Earth Day, etc. A database of such farmers needs to be developed and maintained by the institute. These farmers can be used as key communicators disseminating the technologies developed by the institute.
6. **Agroforestry and Goat Production Business Incubation Centre:** The institute can start an Agroforestry and Goat production Business Incubation Centre for promoting business opportunities and help strengthen the existing value chains. Consultancy services, technology development and commercialization, value addition, facilitating financial and market linkages are some of the extension services that can be provided through this center.
7. **Use of YouTube for information dissemination on scientific practices in agroforestry:** The institute can develop a youtube page exclusively

for disseminating information on scientific practices in agroforestry and success stories. Short length videos can be regularly updated on the youtube channel in the form of demonstration of good agroforestry practices, expert talks on various agroforestry related issues, success stories, panel discussions, etc. It is also important to make use of youtube analytics tool to understand the audience preferences and determinants of video popularity which will help in refining the contents of the videos. Also, content analysis of the comments will help in formulating "frequently asked questions" (FAQs) which can be addressed by the experts, increasing the credibility of information that will help farmers and other stakeholders in making informed decisions.

8. **Use of Poetry, Songs/ Folksongs and Punch lines:** Rural people and farmers show more attention towards poem, songs, folk songs and punch lines for any new idea or message. Therefore, by using agroforestry poems, songs/folksongs, punch lines, etc., dissemination of awareness and creating interest about agroforestry adoption is made easy. For example: poem- Krishivaniki - Ek Jeevan dayini (Agroforestry - A Life giver) (Dwivedi, 2008); Slogan- Lakdi Chara Phal aur Ann - Krishivaniki Hai Jeevan (Wood Fodder Fruit and Grain - Agroforestry Life Again), Ab Ham Sabne Thana Hai- Krishivaniki Apnana Hai (Now we all have decided- Agroforestry has to be Adopted); Song- Krishivaniki Ka Sonu-Sundar Yeh Sandesh, etc.

9. **Krishivaniki sabhas/ Kisan Mela/ Kisan gosthi/Exhibition:** With the joint efforts of the forest department and state agriculture departments *krishivaniki sabhas* can be implemented at village level. Akin to *Karshakasabhas* implemented by the Kerala State Department of Agriculture, these are basically farmers' meet and can be conceptualized as information delivery points where inputs can be seeked from farmers, experts and administrators on local level promotion of agroforestry. Such massive outreach programmes need to be pilot tested for creating better awareness on agroforestry. Also, the success rates of such programmes will be high due to its participatory nature.

10. **Providing incentives to the farmers for promoting agroforestry:** An incentive mechanism needs to be developed to influence the farmers to adopt agroforestry. Reviews suggest three forms of incentives such as market or non-market incentives, regulatory incentives and cross-compliance incentives which influence the adoption of sustainable agriculture practice such as agroforestry. Establishing market linkages, improving the existing market, providing subsidies as seen in *Krushi*

Aranya Protsahana yojana are some of the market incentives while regulatory measures such as trade quotas linked with certification, access to rural credit and crop insurance can play a positive role in adoption rates. Cross-compliance incentives basically includes Payment for Ecosystem Services (PES)/ agri-environment payments which can be made to the farmers for managing their land and providing ecological services. Relaxation on tree regulations to the farmers on tree felling and transportation of timber/non-timber trees if grown on farmers' fields.

11. **Formation of Agroforestry Farmers Producer Organisations (AFPOs):** Forest Producer Organisations are formal or informal associations of indigenous or local people involved in the production, processing and trade of timber and wood products and commercial non-wood forest products (NWFPs). These FPOs may participate in markets for environmental services and carry out different forest-based activities such as representing the interests of small holder producers and influencing the existing policies, collective management of value chains and strengthening the access to markets, leveraging extension and advisory services and capacity building of its members for better knowledge sharing and help in managing natural resources. Tree-grower and agroforestry associations, local community-basedorganizationsassociations of small and medium-sized forest enterprises, associations of indigenous people, associations of community forest enterprises, informal village-level forest management groups, forest owner associations, producer cooperatives and federations of producer organizations are some of the examples of FPOs (FAO and AgriCord, 2016; Pasiecznik and Savenije, 2015).

12. **Creation of ICT based WhatsApp Groups of Targeted Farmers:** ICAR Institutes, CAUs, SAUs, SH&FUs, KVKs, State Line Departments, NABARS and NGOs should create awareness & interest amongst clientele and stakeholders through WhatsApp messaging about agroforestry to bring the benefits of appropriate agroforestry practices to a wider section of the community as well as benefits of livelihood and economic returns for farmers. Time to time messages pertaining to tree, crop and livestock management and weather updates are shared with the group members. Information on organization of extension activities such as agril. exhibitions, kisan mela/kisan gosthi, krishivaniki samachar, prasar patra, extension bulletin, awareness programme is also shared. Video film on different aspect of agroforestry is also shared with the farmers for the management of agroforestry practices. Publications such as folders, bulletins, pamphlets, handouts etc., need to be shared with farmers from time to time.

Conclusion

This article has discussed at length, some of the ICT and extension services that can be adopted to motivate for improving the three phase goat production systems of goat farmers and research workers of agricultural universities and ICAR research institutes and reach the farmers and other stakeholders for up scaling agroforestry activities in our country. It is also important that ICT and extension services need to focus on developing a culture of continuous learning about agroforestry based goat production and the prime focus should be on dissemination of reliable information to the stakeholders. Also, a multi-actor approach engaging a large number of stakeholders need to be adopted for supporting the agroforestry for sustainable goat production system.

References

Dwivedi, R.P. 2015. Per. Communication-Verbatim

Dwivedi, RP. 2008. Poem "Krishivaaniki: Ek Jeevan Daayani" (Agroforestry- A Life Giver) Krishivaniki Aalok. 2008. Vol.2. p-9.

Dwivedi, RP; Kareemulla, K and Rizvi, RH 2013. Agroforestry Systems in Sharanpur and Aligarh Districts of Uttar Pradesh: A Socio-economic Analysis. Indian Journal of Extension Education 49 (3&4): 121-125.

Dwivedi, RP; Tewari, RK; Kareemulla, K; Chaturvedi, OP and Rai, P. 2007. Agri-Horticultural system for household livelihood – A case study. Indian Research Journal of Extension Education 7(1): 22-26.

FAO: 2015. Food & Agricultural Organization of UN http://www.fao.org/forestry/agroforestry/80338/en

FAO and AgriCord. 2016. Forest and farm producer organizations – operating systems for the Sustainable Development Goals (SDGs): strength in numbers. Rome.

Nair, PKR 1989. ICRAF Nairobi Kenya in Leakey, R.R.B. 2017a. Definition of agroforestry revisited. In: Multifunctional Agriculture – Achieving Sustainable Development in Africa, RRB Leakey, 5-6, Academic Press, San Diego, California, USA.

National Agroforestry Policy – 2014 (India) Ministry of Agriculture & Farmers' Welfare, Government of India.

Pasiecznik, N.and Savenije, H., eds. 2015. Effective forest and farm producer organizations. Wageningen, the Netherlands, Tropenbos International.

13

Natural Goat Milk

Satyendra Pal Singh

Rajmata Vijayaraje Scindia Krishi Vishwavidyalaya, Krishi Vigyan Kendra Lahar, (Bhind), Madhya Pradesh

Goats are important components of livestock industry and play a vital role in the socio-economic structure of the economically-week rural community. Goats have been reared as domestic animals across the world. In India, goat keeping constitutes an important business of small and marginal farmers and the landless due to multifold advantages. These are short generation interval, high rate of prolificacy, easy management and marketing as compared to larger ruminants. Goat milk got the nutritional merit of the animal food products in shape of the animal protein. It is highly nutritious, contains essential vitamins and minerals and is an ideal food for the entire family. Though there are 28 registered goat breeds in India (NBAGR, 2017) constituting 26.4 per cent of the world population and are reared very few are having considerable milk producing animal of the country. Goats are highly efficient in converting food stuff, live vegetation, grasses and leaves forage crops, agro-industrial waste and byproducts and even waste cereals unfit for the human consumption to edible milk. Goat milk possesses 19 amino acids in its protein. It has 11 fatty acids in its butter fat, 6 vitamins, 8 enzymes, 25 minerals, 1 sugar, 5 phosphorus compounds, 14 nitrogenous substances all of which are suspended or dissolved in the fluid milk. Goat milk is as close to perfect food as possible in nature. Its chemical structure is amazingly similar to mother's milk. Human infants grow more slowly than the goat kid because the mother milk is low in the protein and calcium needed for the building of the tissues and the bones of the babies. Goats are also maintained as meat animal in India and goat meat represents 0.5 million MT of the total meat produce in the country. India possesses the largest population of goats 135.2 million (19th Livestock census, 2012) that contributes 5 million tons of milk (FAO, 2013). The total production of goat milk also has registered an annual improvement rate of 5.96 percent in India.

Goat Milk

Since ancient time, goat milk has traditionally been known for its medicinal properties, because goats browse on various shrubs and consume leaves and pods of xerophytes trees. The goat milk has recently gained importance in human health due to its proximity to human milk, easy digestibility because of smaller fat globules which makes soft curd. Further it has health promoting traits. Production of goat milk production has increased from 3.34 m MT in 2000 to 5.38 m MT in 2016 (1.6 times) with an annual growth rate of 3.0% India now stand first in goat milk production in the world (The Indian express, March 3, 2016). The top five states in terms of goat milk production are Rajasthan, Uttar Pradesh, Madhya Pradesh, Gujarat and Maharashtra (2014-15). Rajasthan is the leading state in goat milk production with about 1.99 m MT of the 5.05 m MT in the country, which constitutes 36% of the total goat milk produced in the country (GOI, 2016-17).

Table 1: Top Goat Milk Producing States in India

States	Milk Production (000 m MT)	Rank
Rajasthan	1822.82	1st
Uttar Pradesh	1287.84	2nd
Madhya Pradesh	556.75	3rd
Gujarat	267.30	4th
Maharashtra	247.43	5th

Source: Basic Animal Husbandry Statistics, 2014 (BAHS, 2014)

- **Flavor:** Fresh goat milk has a mildly tangy flavor. Due to this off flavor, liquid milk consumption is problematic for children/human and adversely affects its acceptability in society. This flavor is due to the presence of a high proportion of medium chain fatty acids: capric, caprylic and caproic acid. Another reason for the peculiar, strong and undesirable flavor of goat milk may be due to the secretion of hormones by the horns of the bucks. The buck can permeate the milk with its strong musky scent. Moreover, goats are often allowed to consume a variable and improperly monitored feed at any time which also includes improper grazing fields. This can be the cause of off flavor and taste of goat milk.
- **Composition or Nutritional Value:** The composition of goat milk differs greatly from cow, buffalo and human milks (Table 1), and varies with age, breed, individuals, parity, season, feeding, management, environmental conditions, locality, stage of lactation, and health status of the udder (Jenness, 1980). Among the milk components, the fat content varies most (Table 2) in different goat breeds. The wide variations of

major milk constituents' viz. fat and protein content in milk generally affect the biochemical nature, nutritional significance, functionality and utility of goat milk.

Milk is important in the diet because of its protein, calcium and riboflavin content. Protein provides 11 essential amino acids which are deficient in the cereals used for food. Calcium is the nutrient lacking in the diet of those not consuming the milk or milk products. Osteomalacia, osteodystrophy and osteoporosis are the several names of the deficiency symptoms encountered against calcium shortage and diffusion out of the bone. Goat milk proteins are similar to cows but differ in genetic polymorphisms and their frequencies in goat populations. Peptides formed from goat milk casein tastes less bitter than those of cow milk casein. Average amino acid composition of goat and cow milk shows higher levels of six of the 10 essential amino acids: threonine, isoleucine, lysine, cystine, tyrosine and valine.

Table 2: Average Composition of Basic Nutrients in Goat, Sheep, Cow and Human milk

Composition	Goat milk	Sheep	Cow	Human Milk
Fat (%)	3.8	7.9	3.6	4.0
Solid-not-fat (%)	8.9	12.0	9.0	8.9
Lactose (%)	4.1	4.9	4.7	6.9
Protein (%)	3.4	6.2	3.2	1.2
Casein (%)	2.4	4.2	2.6	0.4
Albumin, Globulin (%)	0.6	1.0	0.6	0.7
Non-Protein (%)	0.4	0.8	0.2	0.5
Ash (%)	0.8	0.9	0.7	0.3
Calories/100 ml	70	105	69	68

Table 3: Gross Chemical Composition (%) of Milk of Different Breeds of Goats

Breeds	Water	Total Solid	Fat	SNF	Protein	Casein	Lactose	Ash	Ph
Jamunapuri	86.22	13.78	4.88	8.90	3.85	2.80	4.40	0.85	6.57
Barbari	86.18	13.82	4.86	8.96	4.05	3.10	4.31	0.88	6.58
Beetal	86.38	13.62	4.74	8.88	3.74	-	4.32	0.82	6.59
Sirohi	88.24	11.76	3.58	8.18	-	2.75	-	0.79	6.51
Marwari	87.20	12.80	4.49	8.31	-	2.73	-	0.84	6.50
Kutchi	89.08	10.92	2.99	7.93	-	2.53	-	0.82	6.54
Black Bengal	81.43	18.07	7.93	10.14	4.97	-	4.28	0.89	6.654

Mineral content of goat's milk is much higher than cow or human milk (Table 3). Goat milk contains about 134 mg Ca and 121 mg P/100g, while human milk has only one-fourth to one sixth of these two major minerals. Mineral contents show higher Ca, P, K, Mg, and Cl, and lower Na and S levels than bovine milk. Among trace minerals, both goat and cow milk had more Zn than human milk. Levels of Fe and iodine content in goat and cow milk are significantly higher than in human milk which would be important for human nutrition, since iodine and thyroid hormones are involved in the metabolic rate of physiological body functions. Milk and other dairy products obtained from cows may sometimes interfere with the absorption of Fe from diet. Studies have shown that when goat milk is incorporated into the diet of rats, it produces a greater nutritive use of Fe and minimizes the possible interactions of Fe with other minerals such as Ca, P and Mg, in comparison with animals fed with cow milk.

Table 4: Composition of Goat Milk of Nutritive Value in Comparison with Human Milk

S. No.	Particulars	Per 100 gram		
		Goat	**Cow**	**Human**
1	Total Solids (%)	12.97	12.01	12.50
2	Energy Kilocalories	69	61	70
3	Kilo Joule	288	257	291
4	Protein (%)	3.56	3.29	1.03
5	Lipid (%)	4.14	3.34	4.38
6	Carbohydrate (%)	4.45	4.60	6.89
7	Ash (%)	0.82	0.72	0.20
8	Calcium (mg)	134	119	32
9	Iron (mg)	0.05	0.05	0.03
10	Magnesium (mg)	14	13	03
11	Phosphorus (mg)	121	93	14
12	Potassium (mg)	204	152	51
13	Sodium (mg)	38	49	17
14	Zinc (mg)	0.30	0.38	0.17
15	Ascorbic Acid (mg)	1.29	0.94	5.00
16	Thiamin (mcg)	40	40	20
17	Riboflavin (mg)	0.138	0.168	0.036
18	Niacin (mg)	0.277	0.162	0.036
19	Pantothenic Acid (mg)	0.310	0.314	0.177
20	Vitamin B6 (mcg)	60	60	10
21	Folacin (mcg)	1	6	5
22	Vitamin B12 (mcg)	0.065	0.0357	0.045
23	Vitamin A RE (mcg)	44	52	58
24	Vitamin D (mcg)	0.11	0.03	0.045
25	Vitamin E (mg)	0.03	0.09	0.34
26	Vitamin C (mg)	1	1	4

Cow milk causes some medical problems such as infantile eczema. Many hospitals and medical practitioners in the U.K. keep a list of sources of goat milk that they recommend to patients. The term universal foster mother was often used to describe the goat. Utilization of goat milk can be improved on the advice of medical practitioners for patients suffering from cardiovascular problems, for infant feeds, for nursing mothers and those allergic to cow milk. Goat milk has higher content of monounsaturated (MUFA), polyunsaturated fatty acids (PUFA), and medium chain triglycerides (MCT) than cow milk, which all are proven to be beneficial for human health, especially for cardiovascular conditions. This biomedical superiority has not been promoted much in marketing goat milk, goat yoghurt and goat cheeses, but has great potential in justifying the uniqueness of goat milk in human nutrition and medicine.

Its products are source of protein, phosphate and calcium. The basic nutrient composition of goat milk resembles cow milk, whereas both milks contain substantially higher protein and ash, but lower lactose content. Fat globules are smaller and probably one of the reasons for easy digestion of this milk. There are also differences in the fatty acid profile as goat milk has higher percentage of short and medium-chain (C6-C14) fatty acid.

Characteristics

- Goat milk is alkaline and cow milk is acidic.
- Specific gravity of fresh goat milk 1.026.
- Digestibility coefficient of protein of goat milk is 85%.
- Biological value of goat milk is 87.5%.
- Fat globules are small and fine (size 2 micron) hence it is easily assimilated. Goat milk is naturally homogenized and digested easily.
- The milk does not have gamma-globulin factor.
- Goat milk has 9 minerals more in number than any other milk used for the human consumption.
- The milk protein contains essential amino acids namely arginine, histidine, lysine, isoleucine, valine, trytophane, methioine, threonine and leucine.

Digestibility

Goat milk offers superior digestibility as compared to cow milk. It is generally homogenized and contains greater proportion of fat globules which are easier to digest than cow and buffalo milk. According to the Journal of American Medicine, "Goat's milk is the most complete food known." In fact, the body can digest goat's milk in just 20 minutes, whereas it takes 2-3 hours to digest cow's milk. The superior digestibility of goat milk is due to the following factors:

Size of fat globules

- The fat globules of goat milk are finer than those of cow milk, allowing for a greater surface to volume ratio for enzymatic attack. This enables the fat of goat milk to be broken down and digested more easily.

Presence of Short/Medium Chain Fatty Acid (SCFA/MCFA)

Goat milk is much higher in SCFA and MCFA than cow milk. This means that those SCFA and MCFA have a larger surface-to-volume ratio and are better digestion and absorbed than the long-chain fatty acids (LCFA) prevalent in cow milk. In fact, the levels of the metabolically valuable short and medium-chain fatty acids viz., caproic, caprylic, capric and lauric acids are significantly higher in goat milk and broken down quickly than LCFA of cow milk.

Curd Strength

Goat milk casein forms a less tough and more friable curd than the casein of cow milk. This means the digestive enzymes can break it down more rapidly. As goat milk contains low levels of as_{1-} casein in comparison to cow milk, it produces much softer curd than cow milk.

Presence of Protein-Digesting Enzymes

Goat milk contains proteins that digest in a superior manner. A study investigating the effect of pepsin and trypsin (two protein-digesting enzymes found in the stomach) revealed that while these enzymes completely digested over 96 percent of available goat milk protein, less than 73 percent of available cow milk protein was able to be digested completely. In addition to highly digestible protein, goat milk contains far more digestion-friendly oligosaccharides (prebiotics) than cow milk.

References

FAO (2013). Food and Agriculture Organization.

GOI (2016-17). Government of India.

Jenness, R. (1980). Composition and characteristics of goat milk: review 1968-1979. Journal Dairy Sci. 63: 1605-1630.

NBAGR (2017). National Bureau of Animal Genetic Resources, Karnal (Haryana)

14

Small Ruminant Natural Farming and Export Potential

Anil K. Dixit, Anirudh K.C., Biswajit Sen and Anupam K. Dixit[1]

ICAR-National Dairy Research Institute, Karnal, Haryana
[1]ICAR-Central Institute for Research on Goats, Makhdoom, Uttar Pradesh

Small ruminants (goat and sheep) rearing are considered as natural farming based on two grounds, i.e., (i) their survival on natural resources and are climate resilient, (ii) out of pocket expenses are minimal (Nardone et al., 2004). These animals contributes as livelihood and income augmentation sources for resource poor farmers and immensely contributes by providing milk, meat, fiber, skin, and manure. Goat rearing is done for milk and meat, while sheep is reared mainly for wool and meat purposes and limited use of milk. Goat milk has very high demand globally because of its nutraceutical properties and easy digestibility than bovine milk (Clark et al., 2017), overcome problem of lactose intolerance (Pal et al., 2017), and its nutritionally similarity to human milk (Rai et. al., 2022).

The health benefits of goat milk such as anti-hypertensive, overcome dengue fever, probiotic, antioxidant, antimicrobial properties, and good for gut health are widely recognised by the researchers. The market price of goat milk is almost three times the price of cow milk in different parts of Asia highlighting its income augmentation potential form marginal and small farmers (Liang & Paengkoum, 2019).

Along with raw milk sales, India has an opportunity to expand the processing of goat milk into value-added products which might be highly competent in the international market (Devendra and Liang, 2012). The goat milk products which have export market are: frozen yoghurt, fortified or flavoredmilk, ice cream, butter milk, dried milk or condensed milk product, whey protein concentrate, ghee etc.

The meat of goats and sheep constitutes 13 and 7 percent of total meat production in India. Most of this production is carried out by open grazing and the communities engaged are Bakarwals and Gujjars of Jammu and Kashmir and the Rebari/ Raika groups of western India. Indian sheep milk has very limited use and is used in areas like J & K, Rajasthan, and Gujarat, that too in processed form. Even though wool is an important commodity produced by sheep, due to the lower quality of the wool produced in the majority of the locations except for Jammu and Kashmir, its value is very less when compared to that of traded meat.

India has a promising scope for exporting meat and animal products, considering that its population is vegetarian. Even though Indian meat and by-product export has witnessed high compound growth rates, lack of standardized slaughterhouses, hygiene, cold chain facilities, scattered and unorganized production, and religious constraints have prevented the sector from harnessing its potential (Kumar, 2010; Vidyarthi, 2019). The major sheep-rearing states in the order of population are Telangana, Andhra Pradesh, Karnataka, Rajasthan, Tamil Nadu, Jammu, and Kashmir. Among these states, Telangana and Andhra Pradesh have shown a considerable increase in the size the population from 2012 to 2019 whereas Jammu and Kashmir have recorded a minor decrease in the population. When goat rearing is taken into account, Rajasthan, West Bengal, Uttar Pradesh, Bihar, Madhya Pradesh, and Maharashtra are the major producers (GoM, 2022).

India is the largest exporter of goat and sheep meat in the world with an export of 8696 MT valuing 60.04 million USD in 2021-22 to Qatar, UAE, Kuwait, Maldives, and Saudi Arabia being the major import market for India for the same category (APEDA, 2022). Goats and sheep greatly impact the rural economy mainly due to the ease of production and marketing. Goat and sheep for meat purpose is classified under the HS code 0204.

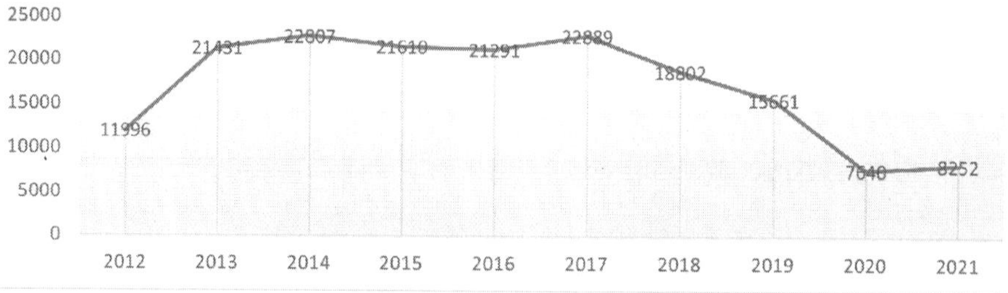

Fig. 1: The export quantity of Indian sheep and goat meat over the years
Source: FAO STAT, 2023

It is evident from Fig. 1 that India's total export of goat and sheep meat was on a rising trend till 2017 and declined in subsequent years. This downfall is mainly attributed due to a decrease in exports to countries such as Saudi

Arabia, Kuwait, UAE, and Qatar as indicated by Fig. 2. The export volume data suggest that India had a fall in the exports made to its loyal partners like Saudi Arabia, UAE, and Qatar. However, Maldives, Oman, and Kuwait have maintained consistency in importing from India.

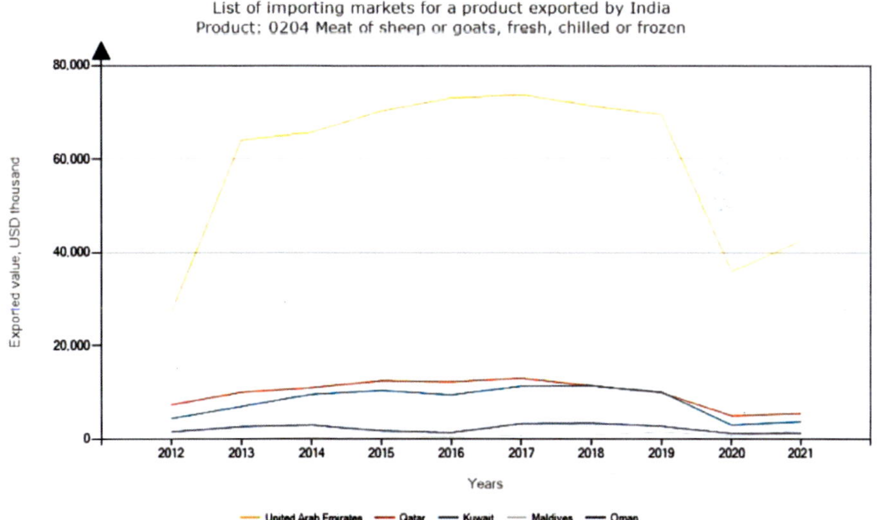

Fig. 2: Export of Indian sheep and goat meat to top five importers over the years
Source: Developed using ITC database

It is very evident from Fig. 2 that the exports to major destinations plateaued for a number of years and dipped during COVID-19 with boundary restrictions. Nonetheless, the trade start gaining momentum with improvement in COVID situation. The main problem with exporting sheep and goats is that there are many nations with tariffs that are comparable to those of our main trading partners, but we are unable to maximise our profits from these nations by expanding our exports to those markets. Figure 4 demonstrates that while certain nations permit Indian beef at low tariffs, our shipments to them are minimal to non-existent. The poor animals management and ineffective value chain is a significant factor in the restricted exports and production (Lata and Mondal, 2021).

It may be noted that these factors stay mostly in India's endeavor to capture the high-end developed markets whereas developing economies in Asia has a preference for low-cost Indian meat. India can gain by directing production in favour of those loyal partners and increasing the volume of trade. Goats and sheep are easy to rear and for the same reason are handled in the highly scattered production system. This sector should be organized through technological interventions and appropriate government support for development of market and value chain infrastructure so as to ensure the trickle-down of benefits to the lower strata. It must also be noticed that the pastures and grazing lands are declining, indicating possible scarcity in green fodder sources from commonly pool resources. The declining common property resources may be a future threat to the rearing of small ruminants. A well-focussed plan is required to maintain and sustain common property resources to support the increasing number of small ruminants.

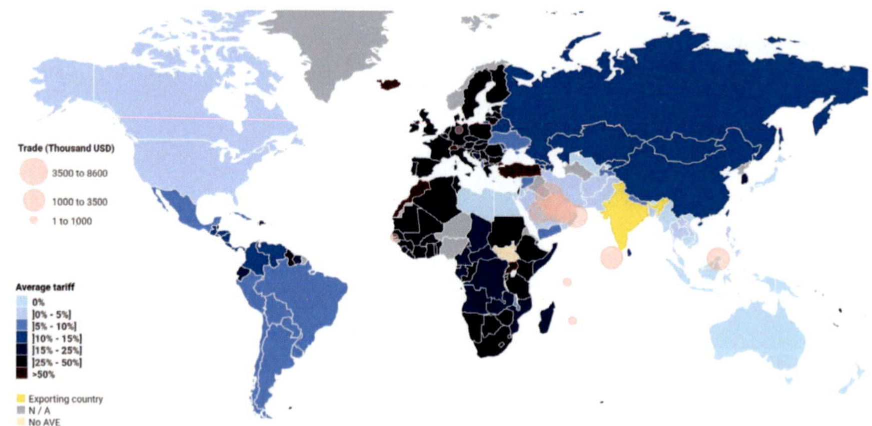

Fig. 3: Tariff and export quantities to different countries (For sheep and goat meat from India)

Export of raw skin/hide of animals is very limited and Nepal is the only consistent buyer of Indian hide. Live animal export is another area related to sheep and goats with UAE, Nepal, Viet Nam, and Maldives being the major importers. Live goats are mainly exported for their meat and religious rituals in particular countries. Live animal export is highly fluctuating. It has to be noted that the fluctuations are mainly caused due to the restrictions on animal exports that are imposed due to the government of India (Manish and Alaudin, 2018). Figure 4 represents the trend in live animal exports from India.

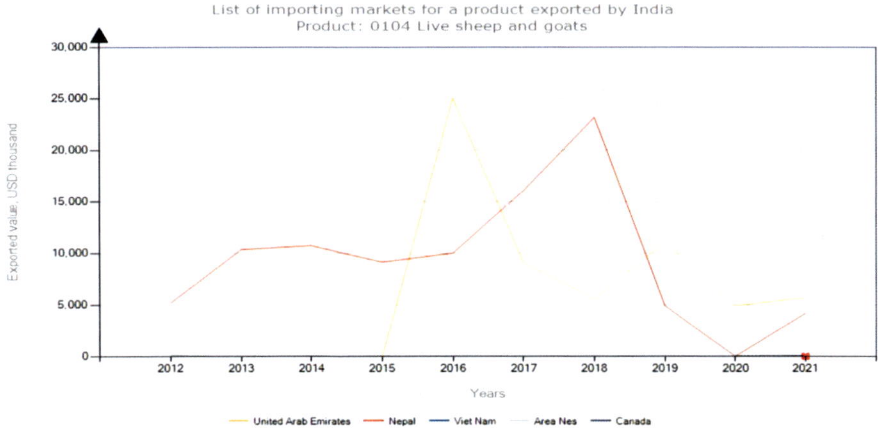

Fig. 4: Export of live sheep and goats from India (HS 0104)

Summary of the Constraints in the Export of Small Ruminants' Products from India

- The majority of the farmers are resource poor, hence the adoption of new technologies is very limited in the sector
- Common property resources are declining which further limits the small ruminants farming
- Lack of access to quality health care and high mortality rates among kids
- Product quality standards and traceability issues
- The lack of marketing infrastructure is another important issue. Most of the goat and sheep herds are maintained in remote areas. The transporting of milk from distant areas, while on migratory route, to collection points is a serious constraint for the farmers
- Synthetic wool is now replacing the natural wool and farmers are not getting the remunerative prices of wool.
- Lack of scientifically maintained slaughterhouses
- Imposition of export restriction on live animals
- Lack of cold chain infrastructure and value chains of meat and milk.

Conclusions

With a proper integration of small ruminant natural farming with processing, marketing and export, this sector can be a boon for less endowed regions of Rajasthan, Uttar Pradesh, M.P., Bihar, West Bengal, Andhra Pradesh, Tamil Nadu, Karnataka, Maharashtra, J &K and north-eastern regions of the country.

References

APEDA. 2023. Sheep and goat meat. Available at: https:https://apeda.gov.in/apedawebsite/SubHead_Products/Sheep_Goat_Meat.htm#:~:text=The%20country%20is%20the%20largest,Maldives%2C%20Saudi%20Arab%2C%20Oman. [Accessed: 13 March 2023].

Clark, S., Garcia, M. B. M. (2017). A 100-year review: Advances in goat milk research. Journal of Dairy Science, 100: 10026-10044.

Devendra, C., & Liang, J. B. (2012). Conference summary of dairy goats in Asia: Current status, multifunctional contribution to food security and potential improvements. Small Ruminant Research, 108(1-3), 1-11.

GoM. 2021. Status of sheep and goat sector of Maharashtra. Available at: http://mahamesh.co.in/en/Menu/SheepAndGoatSectorMaharashtra [Accessed: 13 March 2023].

Kumar, A. (2010). Exports of livestock products from India: Performance, Competitiveness and Determinants. Agricultural Economics Research Review, 23(347-2016-17033), 57-68.

Lata, M., & Mondal, B. C. (2021). Role of goats in Indian economy: Major constraints and routine managemental practices for their wellbeing. Vigyan Varta, 2, 41-46.

Liang, J. B., & Paengkoum, P. (2019). Current status, challenges and the way forward for dairy goat production in Asia–conference summary of dairy goats in Asia. Asian-Australasian Journal of Animal Sciences, 32(8), 1233-1243.

Manish, S & Allaudin, S. "Govt ban on shipping live goats for exports will hurt farmers; here's why". Business Standard, 17 March 2023. P.3

Nardone, A., Zervas, G., & Ronchi, B. (2004). Sustainability of small ruminant organic systems of production. Livestock Production Science, 90(1), 27-39.

Pal, M., Dudhrejiya, T.P., Pinto, S., Brahamani. D., Vijayageetha. V., Reddy, Y. K. & Kate, P. (2017). Goat milk products and their significance, Beverage Food World 44: 21-25

Rai, D.C., Rathaur, A., Yadav. A. K. & Shraddha (2022). Nutritional and nutraceutical properties of goat milk for human health: A review. Indian Journal of Dairy Science, 75(1): 1-10.

Vidyarthi, V. (2019). Trends and Constraints in Export of Animal Products from India. Emerging Global Economic Situation: Impact on Trade and Agribusiness in India, 3.

15

Natural Goat Husbandry Practices in Tripura: Opportunities and Challenges

Asit Chakrabarti[1]* and Vinay Singh[2]

ICAR Research Complex for NEH Region, Tripura Centre, Lembucherra West Tripura, Tripura
[1]Livestock Product Management
[2]Poultry Science

Goat production for milk and meat is an age old practice and goat is one of the first animals to be domesticated by man. Throughout the world goat is considered as 'poor man's cow'. Central Institute for Research on Goats has projected it as 'Future Animal' for rural and urban prosperity (Chakrabarti, 2019). In Switzerland goat is nicknamed as "Swiss baby's foster mother' (Chakrabarti *et al*, 2014). Prasad *et al.*, 2013 opined that among various livestock production enterprises, goat farming is one of the important enterprises, which supports the rural households by providing gainful employment and steady income for the rural masses. The households cultivating less than 2.0 ha of land (marginal and small) are the custodian of more than 76% of the total goats in the country (Singh *et al.*, 2018). The Small ruminants are also important in a diversification strategy that aims to reduce market and climatic risks and optimize the use of available resources (Ayo-Enwerem *et al.*, (2017). Goat farming is an important component in smallholder farming systems in Tripura. Goat rearing has grown from backyard farming to the localized cluster based intensified entrepreneurship activity throughout the state. Goat meat is considered in state is a high value product due to high market price than the any other meat available in the state. Also animals are mostly liked by the native people because of their varied adaptability and presence of lean meat. Goat farming becomes very popular in Tripura because of availability of abundant grass and fodder resources throughout the state. It becomes a significant food source due to its ability to convert poor quality of feed into valuable human food. At present total goat population of the world is more than one billion and 90% are available in developing countries. Asia ranks first in goat population followed by African continent. The total goat population in

India is 148.88 million with an increase rate of 10.1% than the previous census and 20.45% of total livestock population in India. The male goat population is 32.10 million showing a decrease of 14.65%, while female goat population is 116.78 million showing an increase of 19.71% and number of goats in milk is 41.83 million showing an increase of 15.38% over the previous census in India. The Goat population in Tripura is *3.60 lakh* comprising male 51,768 and female 3,08,436. Goat farming in Tripura is a very promising business as the market price of goat meat is Rs.1000 to Rs.1200 per kg. Predominantly Black Bengal and Assam Hill goats are available in Tripura state which is considered as the best quality goat meat breed in the country.

Overview of Tripura State

The Tripura is the third-smallest state with an area of 10,491.69 sq km and population 4.06 million is located in agro-climatic zone of humid Eastern Himalayan Region and situated between 22°56' and 24°32' N latitudes and between 90°09' E and 92°20' E longitudes with an average annual rainfall of 2100 mm. Animal husbandry and agriculture is backbone of the state economy that provides 51% of total workforce in the state. Livestock sector is an indispensible and integral part of agricultural system of the state because of only about 27% of total geographical area available for cultivation and rest 60% is high land (Chakrabarti *et al.*, 2022). The ICAR has categorized Tripura under the Agro-climatic zone of Humid Eastern Himalayan Region. The state has a typical monsoon climate that ranges from sub-tropical in the plains to temperate conditions in hilly areas. Agriculture is the backbone of Tripura's economy that provides employment to nearly 51 per cent of the total work force in the State. Livestock sector is an important part of agricultural system in the state because only about 27% of the total geographical area is available for cultivation and rest 60% is high land.

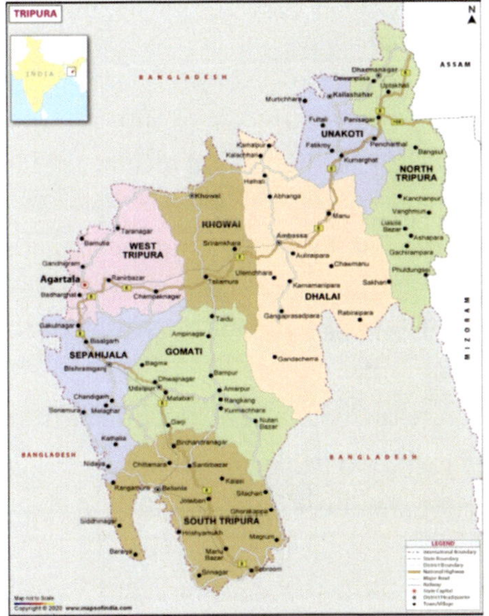

Tripura Map, Source: Internet.

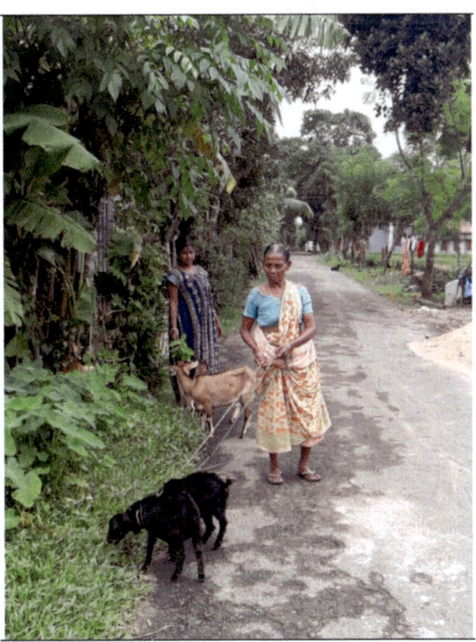

Goat rearing by village women in Tripura

Scope of Livestock Farming in Tripura

In Tripura after agriculture livestock farming is the 2nd most important subsistent activity used to meet household food needs as well as supplement farm incomes. The state is mostly covered with hills; the farmers naturally adopted integrated farming systems for their livelihood. Farmers earns consistent amount of income throughout the year from adoption of integrated farming systems. Due to keen interest of the farmers in livestock rearing, there is huge scope for progressive growth of livestock farming in Tripura. The state also has the potential to adopt organic farming and farmers can earn a good amount of income. As most of the individuals in Tripura prefer eating goat meat, a large numbers of educated youth and entrepreneurs in the recent days show interest in goat husbandry. Recently with the approval of Tripura's first international waterways connecting with river Gomati as Indo-Bangla water route, it has the potential to export and import for livestock component also.

Opportunities of Goat Husbandry in Tripura

1. There is no religious taboo attached with goat farming in Tripura or with goat meat (chevon) and all sections of the society readily consume goat meat.
3. Comparatively low investment is required because of abundant availability of grass and fodder in the state.

4. There is immense scope for starting a small unit of goatery or large commercial farm which suits a small marginal farmer or a big industrialist.
5. In small scale goatery family labour can be efficiently utilized who cannot go for other farming activity (e.g. Children or old member of the family).
6. Due to fastidious eating habit goat can thrive in Tripura climatic condition without any adverse effect.
7. Goat can consume all kinds of plant available in fellow land or in forest and can convert in to valuable animal protein.
8. They are naturally browsing in nature and can easily pluck feed from trees, bushes and shrubs which is readily available in Tripura.
10. Black Bengal or Assam Hill Goats are prolific breeder and mature at the age of 7 to 8 months.
11. Three kidding in two years and twin birth is very common in goats available in Tripura, thus ensure more economic return in a short period.
12. Goat can thrive easily in Tripura and generate employment for rural masses.
13. Its manure is rich in nitrogen, phosphorus and potassium and is excellent low cost manure for agricultural production for small or marginal farmers of the state.
14. Goats are reported to be more economical than cattle and sheep under natural grazing/ browsing (Sharma and Jindal, 2008) and there is a vast scope for natural grazing/ browsing in Tripura.
15. In Tripura goat husbandry has immense importance in agricultural economy through employment and income generation.

Constraints for Goat Husbandry in Tripura

Due to minimum land area of the state, total land area farmers used to face various constraints for goat farming. Such as

1. There is no availability of superior goat germplasm in the state.
2. Land area is very limited for individual farmer.
3. Acute shortage of feed and fodder in the state.
4. Educated youths are not inclining to adopt goat farming.
5. Lack of institutional intervention in encouraging goat rearing.
6. Extension activities are limited to encourage goat farming.

7. Lack of scientific knowledge and scope for fodder cultivation.
8. Due to lack of proper monitoring and timely intervention hampering various goat husbandry projects in the state.
9. Establishment of Entrepreneur for breed development in small ruminant sector e.g. goat farming.
10. Establishment of Regional Semen Production Laboratory and Semen Bank for goat.
11. Import of good goat germplasm from other state or exotic germplasm.
12. Funding of goat of NER with 90:10 ratio.
13. Marketing channels of goats and it products should be properly monitored for better trading.
14. The avenue for export of goat meat or by-products in East and South East Asian countries such as Bangladesh, Myanmar, Bhutan and, China can explored suitably.
15. Proper implementation of livestock policy including goat farming will boost up look east policy of the government.
16. Regular vaccination and treatment is a great constraints for goat farmer of Tripura.

Conclusion

Goat husbandry is a very popular enterprise in Tripura. To boost up the scientific raring of goat and to produce milk, meat and by-products suitable scheme and institutional intervention is urgently necessary for the state. Thus, it will lift up the rural economy of the state as well as it will generate employment at the bottom level. There is vast scope for export import business with surrounding East Asian countries. Establishment of Entrepreneur for breed development in small ruminant sector goat farming is urgently required for the state.

References

Ayo-Enwerem, M.,C., Ahaotu, E. O., Okoro, E.,J. and Nwokocha, V. O. 2017. Voluntary dry matter intake on Panicum maximum and four browse species by West African Dwarf Goats. Proceedings of 42nd Conference, Nigerian Society for Animal Production 26-30 March, 2017. pp. 40-43.

Chakrabarti, A., Godara, R. S., Singh, V. 2022. Pre-weaning growth performance of Black Bengal goat kids in an organized farm in Tripura. The Pharma Innovation Journal 2022; SP-11(6): 2383-2385.

Chakrabarti, A., Kumar, P. R., Mali, S. S., Das, B., Singh, A. K., Bhatt, B. P. 2019. Castrated males a source of extra income from goat rearing in Jharkhand- a case study. Multilogic in Science. Vol. Ix, Issue xxx. 82-84.

Chakrabarti, A., Kumari, R., Dayal, S., Dey, A. 2014 Goat farming- best source of income for rural farmers. Retrieved April 25, 2019, from http://www.krishisewa.com/articles/livestock/406-goatfarming.html.

Chakrabarti A, Daschaudhuri D, Nath K, Das B, Das SP, Das A, et al. National Conference on Agristartups-prospects, Challenges, Technologies and Strategies. 26-27 May, 2022 held at Gangtak, Sikkim.

Prasad, R., Singh, A.K., Singh, L., Singh, A. (2013) Economics of goat farming under traditional low input production system in Utter Pradesh, Indian Research Journal of Extension Education, 13(2): 62-66.

Sharma, M. C. and Jindal, S. K. 2008. Prospects of goat production in India. Compendium of lectures, ICAR sponsored winter school November 25 to December 15, 2008 on Recent advances in improvement of productive and reproductive efficiency of goats through physiological and nutritional interventions, CIRG, Farah, Mathura, U. P.: pp 13-18.

Singh, M. K., Ramachandran, N., Chauhan, M. S., Singh, S. K. 2018. Doubling rural farmers' income through goat farming in India: prospects and potential. Indian Farming 68(01): 75-79.

16

Indigenous Technical Knowledge (ITKS) on Natural Goat Farming

Nitika Sharma, Ashish Srivastava[1], Ashok Kumar Anil Kumar Mishra and A.K. Dixit

ICAR-Central Institute for Research on Goats, Makhdoom, Mathura
[1]College of Veterinary Sciences & Animal Husbandry, U P Pandit Deen Dayal Upadhyaya Pashu Chikitsa Vigyan Vishwavidyalaya Evam Go-Anusandhan Sansthan (DUVASU), Mathura, Uttar Pradesh

The domestication of animals started during Neolithic period. Initially goats and sheep, subsequently cattle and pigs, and lastly draft animals such as horses and asses were domesticated. Thus, goats and sheep were the earliest domesticated animals and rearing of these animals has been centred on food, religion, culture and economy from the ancient times. India's ruminant biodiversity is enriched with 34 breeds of goats (ICAR-NBAGR-2023). At the world level, India ranks second in the goat population and third in sheep population. Even with such impressive genetic resource availability, goat rearing still continues to be a backward profession, primarily in the hands of poor, landless or small and marginal farmers who own either an uneconomical land holding or no land at all. Goats are a source of meat, milk and fibre. The ability of goats to utilize minimal forage, and survive under harsh conditions, makes them a very valuable asset for subsistence farmers. Morbidity and mortality are the two important factors resulting in heavy losses in goat production and improvement programmes. Diseases in goats result in mortality which ranges from 5-25% in adults and 10-40% in kids. In addition, losses due to morbidity result in low productivity. Prevention of disease is always better than cure as it is a lot cheaper. Goat farming is still traditionally oriented and the traditional management systems still hold the key in small ruminant production. Ample information regarding Indigenous Technical Knowledge (ITK) still exists in the farming communities, which helps them in practicing successful goat farming. Even though considerable literature pertaining to treatment of animals using indigenous medicines/herbals is available, references on indigenous husbandry practices in sheep and goat farming are lacking.

Since independence all efforts in India were concentrated on developing an allopathic-based veterinary infrastructure entirely under the government sector. There has been neglect of traditional systems and knowledge to the extent that many of us, even those specializing in veterinary medicine, are unaware of ancient literature and some are even sceptical about it (Rangnekar 1998). In recent years emphasis has shifted towards modern science in the maintenance and development of livestock. With the development of modern medicine, especially after the second world war, traditional medical practices have been increasingly replaced and overlooked at the international level, mostly because many people regarded them as ineffective and useless (Bizimana 1997). Modern medicine was thought to be able to solve almost all health problems of humans and animals. But this overestimation of modern medicine has changed in the course of the 'green wave' since the 1970s, particularly in industrialized countries. The 'green wave' has been characterized by an increasing demand for herbal/ natural products in the form of drugs, food and cosmetics, and was mainly triggered by the side effects resulting from the increasing use of chemicals in various areas of life including medicine. The reconsideration of traditional medicinal systems in the industrialized world and the fact that modern medicine is too expensive for many developing countries were the main reasons for the decision of the World Health Organization (WHO) in the 1970s to promote traditional medicated systems by checking scientifically the efficacy of plants used in traditional medicine and to identify the principles responsible for genuine therapeutic effects (Bizimana 1997).

India, the country of Rishi and Krishi, has a very rich heritage of traditional health management and several treatment systems (Ayurvedic, Unani, Homeopathy) that have been used for animals since time immemorial. These practices have been percolating from one generation to another by oral transmission and considered to be the holistic approach for livestock management methodologies adopted by non-literate cultures. All over India, there are experienced and knowledgeable specialists who practice indigenous techniques but their knowledge is not well documented, merely being transmitted verbally from one generation to the next.

The indigenous technical knowledge (ITK) regarding animal husbandry is considered as old as domestication of various livestock species. Unfortunately, these practices, which are in vogue throughout rural India, are little documented and there is danger of extinction of this knowledge. Thus, it has become imperative to collect and document these practices and to assess their validity.

Under thisbackground, the present paper is an attempt to document the indigenous knowledge prevalent on natural goat farming system. These ITKs collected from different regions of India were found to be effective against many ailments. However, these were perceived to be comparatively less effective than the Modern Veterinary Drug (MVD) in numbers of animals cured and promptness of healing. The Indigenous Practices were perceived better than Modern Veterinary Drugs in respect of their availability, lesser side effects, and lower cost. These Indigenous Practices may be recommended and disseminated among the farmers where MVD is not easily accessible. Moreover these can be blended with modern veterinary drug therapy through laboratory experimentation and scientific validation.

Disease/ condition	**ITKs Used**
Wound	• Sap extracted from leaves of Grihtkumari (Scientific name: *Aloe barbadensis*) to be applied topically. Also effective in burns and injuries caused due to fire. • Sap extracted from leaves and stem of Kesurta (*Scientific name: Scirpus grossus*) is mixed with *Lahsun* (English name:Garlic,Scientific name: *Allium sativum*) and to be applied topically. • *Haldi* (English name: Turmeric, Scientific name: *Curcuma domestica*) is grounded and applied topically. • Extract of *Gainda* (English name: African marigold, Scientific name: *Targetes erecta*) leaves is applied topically. • *Jiyeti* plant is to be burnt and ash of *Jiyeti* is then mixed with coconut oil and applied topically. • Extract of *Bisalyakarani* (Hindi name: *Ghamra;* Scientific name: *Tridax procumbens)* leaves is applied topically. • Powder is made by grinding the seeds of *Sharifa* (English name: Custard apple, *Annona squamosa*) and applied topically on the worm-infested wound. • Paste is made from root, bark of *Jamun* (Scientific name: *Syzgium jambolanum*) and applied topically on wound. • Fruits of *Khudikathi* are to be grounded and mixed with coconut oil and applied topically. • Roots of *Kuchila* (English name: Snakewood, Scientific name: *Strychnos nux-vomica*) and roots of *Surjamukhi* (English name: Common sunflower, Scientific name: *Helianthus annuus*) is mixed with *Palas* (Scientific name: *Butea monosperma*) petals and mustard oil and applied topically over the wound. • Latex of *Akanda* (Hindi name: Madar, Family: Asclepiadaceae, Scientific name: *Calotropis gigantica*) is applied topically.
Bloat	• Ten gram *Amla* (Scientific name: *Emblica officinalis*), 10 gram *Haritaki* (Scientific name: *Terminalia chebula*) and 10 gram *Bahera* (Scientific name: *Terminalia bellirica*) are mixed and fed to the animal daily once for 7 days. • Ten gram bark of *Aswatha* (English name: Banyan, Scientific name: *Fiscus benghalensis*), 10 gram *Adrak* (Ginger, Scientific name: *Zingiber officinale*) and 10 g salt are mixed and fed to the goat daily once for 7days.

Disease/ condition	ITKs Used
	• Twenty ml sap extracted from leaves of *Kadam* (Scientific name: *Anthrocephalus cadamba*) is drenched to the goat for 2-3 days. • Mixture of 50 gram *Somraj* (Scientific name: *Centrathierum anthelminticum*) and 20 gram *Indrajan* (English name: indigo plant, Scientific name: *Wrightia tinctoria)* is fed to the goat. • Twenty ml decoction of stem bark of *Kadam* (Scientific name: *Anthocephalus cadamba*) is given to the animal.
Diarrhoea	• Pulp of 100 gram old ripened *Imli* (Tamarind, Scientific name: *Tamarindus indica*) is fed to the animal for two to three days. • Fifty ml sap of *Amrood* (English name: Common guava,Scientific name: *Psidium guajava*) leaves is fed. It is efficient especially for goat. (Srivastava et al., 2016) • Juice of *Anarash* (English name: Pine apple, Scientific name: *Ananus comosus*) leaves is mixed with water and then is to be drenched 100 ml daily for 2-3 days. • *Rakta Kambal* leaves (English name: Indian red water lily, *Nymphaea nouchali*) are mixed with soda and then fed to the goat, 10 ml daily for 2-3 days when it is suffering from blood mixed diarrhoea. • Sap of 50 ml *Kela* (English name: Edible banana, Scientific name: *Musa paradisiaca*) leaves and 20 ml sap of *Bans* leaves (English name: Bamboo, Scientific name: *Bambusa arundinacea*) are mixed with 50 gram sugar and fed to the goat for 2-3 days. • Bark and fruits of *Bahera* tree (Scientific name: *Terminalia bellirica*) are pulverised and mixed with water then it is boiled and to be fed 10 ml every day for 4-5 days. • Ten ml sap of *Imli* (English name: Tamarind, Scientific name: *Tamarindus indica*) leaves and *Sonal* leaves are mixed with *Kali mirch* (English name: Black pepper, Scientific name: *Piper nigrum)* and then given orally for 3-4 days. • Twenty ml sap of *Kurchi* (Scientific name: *Holarrhaena antidysenterica*) leaves is to be fed to the cattle for 2-3 days. (Sharma et al., 2022) • Ten ml Juice obtained from bark of *Sal* tree (Scientific name: *Shorea robusta*) and then it is to be drenched. • Ten to twelve ml decoction of stem-bark of *Khair* (English name: Cutch tree, Scientific name: *Acacia catechu*) is given to the animal twice daily for 2-3 days.
Dysentery	• One hundred to one hundred fifty gram *stem*, leaves of *Anantamul* (English name: Indian sarsaparila, Scientific name: *Hemidesmus indicus*) is grounded and juice is extracted and mixed with honey and to be fed to the animal suffering from dysentery. • Three pieces of *Kalimirch* (English name: Black pepper, Scientific name: Piper nigrum) *Liquorice* (Scientific name: *Glcyrrhiza glabra*), 2 teaspoon full ghee and 10 gram smashed *Jastimadhu* are mixed with 50 ml cold water and to be drenched.

Disease/ condition	ITKs Used
	• Ten ml extract of *Gainda* (English name: African marigold, Scientific name: *Targetes erecta*) shoot is mixed with 10 ml extract of *Durba* (Hindi name: Dhub grass, Scientific name: *Cynodon dactylon)* and is drenched to the animal. • Three pieces of *Kali mirch* (Black pepper, *Piper nigrum*), 5 gram ajawain (English name: *Bishop's weed*, Scientific name: *Trachyspermum ammi*) and 5 gram *Chirata* (Scientific name: *Folia varpulchella*) are grounded and fed to the animal for 3-4 days. • Bark of *Palas* tree (Scientific name: *Butea monosperma*) is boiled with 50 ml water and then is drenched to the goat for 3-4 days. • Forty gram *Kalmegh* (Creat, Scientific name: *Andrographis paniculata*) leaves and 20 gram *Thankuni* leaves (Indian pennywort, Scientific name: *Centella asiatica*) are grounded to make a paste and then fed to the cattle. • One hundred ml extract of *Kurchi* (Scientific name: *Holarrhena antidysenterica*) leaves is drenched to the animal for 2-3 days.(Sharma et al., 2022) • Decoction of the root of *Babul* (Scientific name: *Acacia arabica*) is mixed with mustard oil in the ratio of 1:3 and to be drenched to the animal.
Arthritis	• Decoction of the root of *Babul* (Scientific name: *Acacia arabica*) is mixed with mustard oil in the ratio of 1:3 and to be drenched to the animal. • Hot fomentation is given with *Akanda* leaves (Hindi name: *madar* Asclepiadaceae, Scientific name: *Calolropis gigantean;*) along with ghee. • A luke warm paste is made from *Lahsun* (English name: Garlic, Scientific name: *Allium sativum*) and ghee and applied on the affected part.
Cough and cold	• Twenty gram *Tulsi* leaves (English name: Holy basil, Scientific name: *Ocimum sanctum*) and 20 gram *Basak* leaves (Scientific name: *Adhatoda vasica*) are boiled with water. Then extracted juice is mixed with 1-teaspoon honey and fed to the animal. • Three to four pieces of *Tejpata* (Scientific name: *Cinnamomum tamala*), 10 gram *Adarak* (English name: Ginger, Scientific name: *Zingiber officinale*) and *Pipal* (Scientific name: *Ficus religiosa*) leaves are mixed. Extract is made from the mixture and is drenched to the animal along with water. • Efflorcence of *Tulsi* (English name: Holy basil, Scientific name: *Ocimum sanctum*) and *Basak* (Scientific name: *Adhatoda vasica*) leaves are mixed and extract is taken and mixed with ghee, *Adarak* (Ginger,Scientific name: *Zingiber officinale*) and molasses and fed to the goat. • A paste is made from ghee, *Kali mirch* (English name: Black pepper, Scientific name: *Piper nigrum*), *Adarak* (English name: Ginger, Scientific name: *Zingiber officinale*) and *Lahsun* (English name: garlic, Scientific name: *Allium sativum*). Then it is divided into 2 parts. One part is fed to the animal and other part is topically applied over head and neck.
Intestinal worms	• Red powder obtained from surface of the fruits of (Scientific name: *Mallotus philippensis)* (Kamala, Raini) can be fed orally to remove the threadworms and Ascaris. • Root of *Garanda* (Scientific name: *Carissa caranta)* can be mixed with pericarp of mango (Scientific name: *Mangifera indica* L. Anacadiaceae) in water and used as oral antihelmintic.

Disease/ condition	ITKs Used
	• The decoction of root and leaves of neem can be given orally to goats for elimination of intestinal worms as anthelmintic. • Pumpkin seed, black walnut, garlic, wormwood, wild mustard, wild carrots, etc. act as vermifuge.
Ticks/ lice infestation	• Boil 50 grams of Tobacco (Scientific name: Nicotiana tabacum) leaves in 800 ml of water. Add just enough soap (around 50 gram) to cause a little foaming. Wash or spray the affected animals with this liquid.
Poisoning	• Grind the charcoal 200gram and mix it with 800 ml of fresh milk and 400ml of water. Drench 1.2 litres of the mixture to adult goat at one time and 600ml to kids.
For increasing milk production	• '*Pinda'* a local feed prepared by mixing wheat flour in lukewarm water with *Jaggery* (*Gur)*, butter (extracted from curd), rice, *Jhingora* (Scientific name: *Echinochola frumentacea*), *Bhimal'(*Scientific name: *Grewia optiva)*leaves, Bhatt (black Soybean), *Binola* (cotton seeds), *Methi* seeds and *Dhalia* (broken wheat). • The stem along with leaves of bhimal or bihul (Scientific name: *Grewia optiva)* is cut periodically and fed to milch/ lactating animals

References

Acharya RM. Sheep and Goat Breeds of India. FAO Animal Production and Health Paper-30, FAO ROME; 1982.

Bizimana Nseknye 1997Scientific evidence of efficacy of medicinal plants for animal treatment, Ethno veterinary Medicine: Alternatives for Livestock Development, Proceedings of an International Conference held in Pune, 4-6 November, **2:** Abstracts, pp. 11-12.

Burman, RR, Singh SK. Indigenous tech knowledge component in participatory research. Agriculture Extension Review. 2005; 17(3):24–30. 106

Government of India. Planning Commission Report, New Delhi; 2007.

ICAR-NBAGR-2023. Available from: https://nbagr.icar.gov.in/en/registered-goat/

Immanuel RR, Imayavaramban V, Elizabeth LL, Kannan T, Murugan G. Traditional farming knowledge on Agroecosystem Conservation in Northeast Coastal Tamil Nadu. Indian Journal of Traditional Knowledge. 2010; 9(2): 366–74.

Rangnekar D V 1998Random thoughts on Ethno veterinary Practices and their Validation in relation to Livestock Development in India, ICAR short course entitled "Techniques for scientific validation and Evaluation of Ethno veterinary practices" pp. 24-27.

Soundararajan C, Palanidorai R, Sivakumar T. Efficacy of tamarind seed coat powder against Cutaneous Myiasis in Sheep, Goat and Pig. In: Compendium released during International Conference on EthnoVeterinary Practices, 2010 Jan 4–6, TANUVAS, VUTRC, Thanjavur, India; 2010. p. 140

Sharma, N., Mishra, A.K., Kumar, A., Srivastava, A., Gururaj, K., Singh, D.D, Singh, T.P and Pawaiya, R.V.S.2022. Antibacterial activity of traditionally used plants against the resistant enteropathogenic Escherichia coli. Indian J. Animal Res., 56(6):759-763. DOI:10.18805/IJAR.B-4844.

Srivastava, A. and Mondal, D.B.2016. Comparative evaluation of antibacterial efficacy of plants traditionally used as antidiarrheal against enteropathogenic Escherichia coli. Indian J. Animal Res., 50:80-84.

17

Present Scenario and Opportunities in Goat Farming in Madhya Pradesh

S.C. Srivastava, J.S. Rajput and Raj Singh Kushwah

Rajmata Vijayaraje Scindia Krishi Vishwa Vidyalaya, Krishi Vigyan Kendra Gwalior, Madhya Pradesh

The livelihood in rural India mainly depends on agriculture in the form of various land-based enterprises like crop farming, livestock rearing etc. But the landless people in the villages depend mainly on agricultural wages. These landless rural resource poor possess own labour as the only abundant factor which is free to them and they try to use it to its maximum for their survival and thus concentrate on animal husbandry. Goats are kept as a source of additional income and as an insurance against income shocks of crop failure. In addition, the rural poor who cannot afford to maintain a cow or a buffalo find goat as the best alternative source of supplementary income and milk. Goats represent a more liquid form of capital than cattle and are readily tradable, hence goats are called as "poor man's cow" in Indiabecause it will produce milk, meat and manure like cow at very low costs.Goats are also perceived to be a less risky to invest into compared to sheep. Goat rearing has significant effect in augmenting farmers' income. Goats preferentially select plant parts that are higher in digestibility when stocking density is low. Tolerance of goats toward bitterness may play an important role in maximizing grazing capacity and in biological control of weeds. Goats will sustain and produce well under low fodder, low water and extreme adverse climate and it will produce well in terms of milk, meat, manure and hide. Goats are docile, good tempered, cooperative animals easy to rear by women, land less labour and children and they will thrive well on shrubs, bushes and kitchen waste. They are known as moving ATM because they will provide financial assistance to farmer thought the year in all situations.

Goat is the one of the early domesticated animal, earlier goat farming activity was limited to livelihood activity, now it become as a important commercial activity. As per 20th livestock census,India has 148.88 million goats population, which is second largest in the world. 70 million farmers of over 5 Lakhs remote villages of India involved in the goat farming business. 70 percentage of goats In India reared by landless labourers, marginal farmers and nomads

India is the largest goat milk producer in the world, followed by Bangladesh (2.2 million MT) and Sudan (1.5 million MT).China produces about 1.8 million MT meat (highest in world), followed by India (0.5 million MT) and third is Nigeria (0.3 million MT). In India, goat sector contribute about 14,453 crores, out of which 6851 crore from meat, 4588 crores from milk and 648 crores from skin, which is 8% of total GDP from livestock sector and generate 4% employment directly or indirectly in the country. Approximately 20 million small and marginal farmers depend on goat rearing. The industrialized country with the biggest appetite for goat is China, with 3.5 pounds eaten per capita each year. Depending on your family's heritage and the part of the country in which you live, you might have more than a passing familiarity with goat meat

Madhya Pradesh is one of the biggest state in India with lots of trees and shrubs .There are lots of scope for goat farming as there is plenty green fodder is available there is a huge demand for goat meat than sheep meat in Madhya Pradesh there are many commercial goat farming and goat breeding centres available in Madhya Pradesh you get cheap labour for managing your goat farm Establishing and managing goat farming in Madhya Pradesh is not that hard task god is considered a poor mans cow in India and very well suited for the dryland farming system. Goat farming can be established in areas where marginal or undulating lands are available. In Madhya Pradesh goats can be reared for milk, meat fibre and skin. Commercial goat farming in Madhya Pradesh can also fetch additional income since goats can produce manure Stall-Fed goat farmers can practice the extensive rearing method provided there is enough grazing land in their local area In upcoming sections let us talk more about goat farming advantages in Madhya Pradesh goat faming care in Madhya Pradesh goat breeds in Madhya Pradesh there are subsidies and loans available under various schemes for Goat Farming in Madhya Pradesh.

Advantage of Goat Farming in Madhya Pradesh

- Madhya Pradesh state has vast agricultural grazing lands for goat farming so going for goat farming in the state is very easy.
- **Very low investment:** in the cost of one pregnant buffalo we can get 10 pregnant goats.
- Compared to other states, labour in Madhya Pradesh is cheap for managing goat farming

- Goats are friendly and multipurpose animals that can be raised along worth other animals.
- One can earn profits with goat farming by selling meat, milk, fibre, skin, and manure.
- **Less labour requirement:**Under grazing system 30-40 goats and under stall feeding 40-80 goats can be reared by single person. Compared to other animal farming goat farming needs less lobourers.
- **Multipurpose animal**: Goat will produce milk, meat, skin, manure and kids.
- **High prolificacy**: goat has extraordinary reproductive ability compared to other domestic animal species, yearly twice kidding and twin and triplets are common in goats.
- **Easy to rear**: they will not demand high profile nutrition, they will survive and reproduce with low quality feed and fodder.
- Goats are hardy animals and can survive any kind of climatic conditions in Madhya Pradesh.
- Chevon contains low cholesterol and a lean meat than red meat.
- According to availability of land, labour and capital the goatery can be started with one unit of goat to a large commercial farm which suits a small marginal farmer or a big industrialist.
- In small scale goatery family labour can be efficiently utilized who cannot go for other farming activity (e.g. Children or old member of the family).
- Due to fastidious eating habit goat can thrive in all agro-climatic condition of the country.
- Goat can consume all kinds of plant which are generally rejected by the other animals and also can withstand more bitter taste.
- Due to small fat globule present in goat milk, it is easily digested and medically recommended for infants and aged people.
- Goats are prolific breeder and mature at the age of 10 to 12 months. In small breeds like Black Bengal or Assam Hill it is only 6 to 7 months. By 16 to 17 months goats starts milking.
- Three kidding in two years and twin birth is very common in goat, thus ensure more economic return in a short period.
- Goat manure is rich in nitrogen, phosphorus and potassium and is excellent manure for agricultural production.

- Goats require less maintenance and low inputs the setup cost and feed requirement are less compared to other livestock businesses.
- Goat meat is considered lean meat and a good source of protein No need to have special skills in marketing Goat meat is tasty and has excellent demand in Madhya Pradesh and surrounding states In India.
- Goat milk is highly nutritious, having more solids, easily digestible and less allergic compared to other species. Goat milk is also used in the preparation of ayurvedic medicines.
- Goat manure has 2.5 times more nitrogen and phosphorus compared to cattle and buffalo manure, so agriculture and horticulture farmers have more faith on goat manure.
- Goats are hardy livestock and they have very good disease resistance capacity.
- Goat farming set up in Madhya Pradesh is very easy and even women and older people can maintain the daily activities in the farm.
- You can choose airy goat farming as well if u finds the right market for goat milk in Madhya Pradesh you can get excellent profits goat milk is better than cow milk in terms of digestion.
- Nowadays many people are showing interest in setting up a goat farming business in Madhya Pradesh to support the local employment and lift them from the poverty line.Unemployed people in Madhya Pradesh, who are interested to earn part-time or full-time considering goat farming business as their livelihood.
- Goats can produce more than one kid in a single birth, depending on breed. Hence, one can expect more goats in a short period of time.
- In case if u are not able to set up a commercial scale, you can raise the goas as pets in your backyard to earn some of your family expenses.
- Goats can help in small cleaning plants, leaves, shrubs, and weeds apart from this, goat manure is very useful for growing agricultural crops.
- You can sell goat manure or can use it to grow fodder cropsthis can reduce feed costs drastically.
- The goat skin has excellent demand in Madhya Pradesh as the quality of goat skin is good.
- Compared to other livestock, goat have early reproduction and less gestation period
- The goat farming business is proven and successful so u should not have a second thought about starting a goat farm in Madhya Pradesh.

- Goat farming requires less labour you can run the farm with seasonal labour.
- The space requirement depends on the number of goats usually goats do not require much floor space in the shed/goat house you don't need and expensive goat house.

Goat Farming Systems in Madhya Pradesh

1. Zero grazing (Intensive) goat farming system: in this type of goat farming system, the animals are not allowed outside for grazing on green pastures. Goats are reared by feeding in the goat house itself. This method of rearing is also called intensive stall-fed goat farming.
2. Semi grazing (Intensive) goat farming system: in this farming method, goats are allowed to free-range grazing for some time, then they return to the goat house. They are fed in the goat house for the remaining of the day.
3. Extensive goat farming system: in this farming system, goat are allowed in free-range grazing for a whole day and they allowed in the house at night for resting.

Constraints in Goat Farming

- Unavailability of high genetic potential breeds of goat.
- Absence of high producing exotic cross breed.
- Lack of scientific feeding practices and feeding management at farmer level.
- Buying unhealthy goats.
- Lack of proper training.
- Getting too many goats too fast.
- Insufficient knowledge.
- Failure to choose the right breed.
- Numerous breeds are available.
- Ignoring mineral needs.
- Research your market before buying your first goat.

Challenges in goat farming: Challenges includes, highly unorganized and most of time monopoly marketing, Endemic disease problems, limited feed resources due to farmers are behind the commercial crop practices, due to urbanization and industrialization grazing land of goats depleting every year. Water problem due to low rain, climatic variations like famine, flood and lightening strike and labour shortage. Unavailability of high genetic potential breeds of goat, absence of high producing exotic cross breed, lack of scientific feeding practices and feeding management at farmer level. High kid mortality due to colibacillosis starvation, extreme climatic condition, death of mother due to parasitic infestation as a result of poor management.

Challenges can be overcome by change in marketing strategy, growing of fodder crops and trees, conservation and harvesting of rain water, following of alert message about climatic variations, practicing hygiene in the goat she and regular following of deworming, dipping for external parasites and vaccination schedule and good management practices in the farm will reduce the kid and adult mortality in the farm.

Marketing of goat: Marketing is the challenging task in goat farming. Most of time farmer and butcher will get same margin. Farmer's faces monopoly systems due to butchers are the only buyers. For better returns and profit sell goat milk and meat directly to consumers. Selling to new farming units or new farmers who are starting goat farming will have good margin. Don't farm high profile breeds for local butchers because they will purchase at low rate leads to loss and high profile breeds needs more care and feed inputs leading to increase cost of production. Start farming with local breeds updates the market and once you get good market than update your breed in the farm. Create a market channel in cities for milk and meat. Sell the goats during peak demand situations like bakrid, dashara, village festival seasons where there is a huge demand for goats especially male goats. Recently male kid rearing in goat becoming popular due to short period of rearing of male kids having more demand and farmers will get more margin in terms of rupees. Milk more demand in cities-100 ml, 200 ml, 500 ml. Make an arrangement with corporate companies for the sale of milk and meat in cities for competitive price.

Tips for Successful Goat Management

1. Follow regular deworming and vaccination, don't wait for disease to come.
2. For local market local breed of goat are best.
3. Start farming with the guidance of veterinarian.
4. Don't rear grazing goats install feeding farms and vice versa.
5. Semi intensive farming is the best method for the goat farming.
6. Start farming with local breeds and create your own market channel for milk and meat, than upgrade your breeds in the farm.

7. Regular hygiene and good management practices are very much essential for optimum production.
8. Work in already running goat farms for a period of 15 days to one month before starting your goat farming unit.
9. Visit nearby local livestock market and have an idea about goat deman, supply and market.
10. Seasonal management is essential for better performance.
11. Isolation and prompt treatment is very much essential for control of disease.
12. Cultivation of fodder and fodder plants are key to success in goat farming.
13. Feeding of low amount of concentrate and high amount of roughages will be ideal for goat feeding.
14. Provide regular clean and fresh drinking water and urea molases blocks licking will enhances the production of saliva and there by improves the digestion in goats.
15. Foot baths and applying of lime powder in rainy season will reduce the foot rot incidence in the farm.
16. Proper collection and sell of goat manure will increase the income of goat farming.
17. Sale of goats in the high demand seasons like bakrid, dashara and village festival will have more income compared to sale in lean season.
18. Have infestation and affinity towards animals.
19. Regular animal health check up should be done for control of diseases.
20. Restrict unauthorized movement of animals and human in the goat farm.

18

Natural Goat Production in Gujarat Economic Analysis

Narendra Singh and A.K. Dixit[1]

NAUA&T, Navsari, Gujarat
[1]ICAR- Central Institute for Research on Goat, Mathura, Uttar Pradesh

Among the small ruminants, goat is perhaps the most useful animal providing milk as well as meat. It is also superior in converting the feeds to meat and other products in a short period than most of the other livestock (Pandit&Dhaka,2005). Goats contribute milk, meat, fiber, skins and manure to the subsistence of small holders and landless rural poor. Goat meat accounted for almost 37 per cent of the total meat production in the country (Chandra, 2002). Importance of goats lies in the fact that human population is increasing very rapidly creating increasing demands for animal protein foods on the one hand and the feed resources for large ruminants are decreasing due to shrinkage of grazing lands on the other.Goats make important economic contributions in India. They are so vital to a large human population that their contribution to national economy cannot be overlooked. Goats require relatively much lower investments and facilities in terms of housing, feed, labour and health care. There is quick pay of dues because of fast multiplication and early maturity. Further, the risk involved in goat farming is much lower compared to other livestock and crops production.In Gujarat state, Population of milch goat has shown increasing trend as it was 23.36 lakh in 1951 and in year 2019 it found 48.68 lakh, which shows 47.98%, increased. As per the previous livestock census i.e. 2012, goat population declined by 1.84 percent which shows goat farming should give emphasis to enhance rural farmer's income.

India has a very large and diverse genetic resource of goats. Goat plays a significant role in economic upliftment of rural poor of our country. Consumption of goat meat (chevon) is increasing rapidly due to its social acceptability. This sector has tremendous potential in employment generation & poverty reduction.

Goats are among the main meat-producing animals in India, whose meat (chevon) is one of the choicest meats and has huge domestic demand. Due to its good economic prospects, goat rearing under intensive and semi-intensive system for commercial production has been gaining momentum for the past couple of years. High demand for goat and its products with potential of good economic returns have been deriving many progressive farmers, businessmen, professionals, ex-servicemen and educated youths to take up the goat enterprise on a commercial scale. The emerging favourable market conditions and easy accessibility to improved goat technologies are also catching the attention of entrepreneurs. A number of commercial goat farms have been established in different regions of the country. The study was undertaken to study economics and value chain analysis of goat farming and role of goat farming in sustainable farmers income.

Data and Methodology

The study was conducted in South Gujarat region which comprises of seven districts viz: Navsari, Valsad, Bharuch, Surat, Narmada, Tapi and Dang. Among these seven districts, Navsari, Valsad and Tapi districts were purposively selected for the present study. These districts possess 43% of total goat population of the state (Govt of Gujarat, 2021-22). Multistage stratified random sampling technique was used for the study. There are 15 talukas in these districts out of which six talukas and 18 villages were selected randomly. First of all the list of goat keepers was prepared in the selected villages. Then the whole list was divided into surati and local breed goat keepers. The goat keepers in the selected villages were categorized on the basis of their herd size groups as Small (1 to 5 goats, kids & buck), Medium (6 to 15 goats, kids & buck) and Large (16 to or more goats, kids & buck).

The study covered 180 goat keepers in all, consisting of 15 goat keepers in small, 20 in medium and 7 in large group from surati breed and 67 in small, 57 in medium and 14 in large group of local breed of goats. These were selected on the basis of probability proportionate to the number of households in each category. The data for the study were collected through a well structured pre-tested schedule by personal interview method. The statistical means like means and percentage were used to analyze the data.

Results and Discussion

The results of study were divided into three parts: (a) Distribution of goats per households and (b) Economics of goats farming (c) Value chain analysis of goat marketing.

(a) **Distribution of goats**: The number of goats (with buck & kid) belonging to surati and local breed per household owned by different herd size groups has been shown in Table 1. The total number of goats was higher in local breed (2843) than surati breed (793). From the Table-1 it could be observed that the goat keepers keep more local breedable bucks than surati goat keepers.

Table 1: Distribution of goat per house hold

Particulars	Surati				Local				Grand Total
	Small	Medium	Large	Total	Small	Medium	Large	Total	
No. of Breeding Male/Buck	8	26	22	56	64	104	44	212	268
No. of Lacting/ breed able female (>1yr)	62	289	260	611	610	1073	497	2180	2791
Kids & Adult up to 12 month	10	54	62	126	109	242	100	451	577
Male	4	16	17	37	28	69	29	126	163
Female	6	38	45	89	81	173	71	325	414
Total Strength	80	369	344	793	783	1419	641	2843	3636

Economics of goat farming:A comparative economics of goat farming for different herd size of surati and local goats worked out, as shown in Table 2. The total expenditure of goat farming was divided into various components like value of existing stock, cost of feed, cost of labour, value of shed, miscellaneous cost & veterinary expenses and interest on total expenditure. The annual total expenditure per goat per year was worked out as INR 5521.76 for small herd size group, INR 4932.62 for medium herd size group and INR 4580.67 for large herd size group in surati goats. While in local goats, the total expenditure per goat per year was INR 4706.30 for small herd size group, INR 4080.09 for medium herd size group and INR 3853.88 for large herd size group. Thus, the total expenditure was higher in surati goats than the local goats. Except labour, expenditure incurred on cost of feed was nearly 14.45 per cent in surati breed and 11.82 per cent in local breed. The explanations of low feed cost of goat farming in both breeds of goats were reared under extensive system of management. Ahir community found in valsad district usually use grazing practices on nearby forest area which reduces cost of feeding. They use 6 to 8 hours grazing daily throughout the year. Similar observation was made by Singh *etal.*(2011).

The expenditure incurred on cost of labour use was 22.28 per cent in surati breed and 25.17 per cent in local breed. The goat keepers, use labours due to this cost was not paid in both of breed because where every time use in spare family labour even children and woman.

Returns in the goat farming include value of milk, sale of kids & goats and value of manure. The annual net income per goat was observed to be substantially higher in surati breeds. It was INR 922.74, INR 1209.90 and INR 1446.36for small, medium and large herd size groups respectively, in surati breed, while in case of local breed for the respective herds of goat farming were in comparatively less. The possible explanation for higher net income among surati breed was due to sale of milk, better management practices for surati goat. The overall average net income was INR 1283.51 in case of surati breed and INR 994.90 in case of local breed this was due to relatively lower cost of goat farming. The results are comparable with earlier studies under field condition (Bhatia *et al., 2005*Palanichamy *et al.,* 2007 & Tyagi *et al.,*2013)

Value Chain Analysis of Goat Marketing

The marketing of livestock in general, and of goats in particular, in India is not orderly and efficient. There are a number of marketing channels and several market intermediaries are involved in a particular marketing channel.

Therefore, the producer is usually deprived of his due share in the buyer's rupee. Although some studies as those by Dixit and Shukla (1995), Shukla *et al.*(1996), Singh and Hussain (1996) and Kumar and Singh (1999) & Pandit & Dhaka,2005, have been made on goat marketing. The marketing of goats has been studied in the nearby sachin market which is run by Surat municipal corporation. Data have been collected from 25 sellers and 25 buyers, selected randomly from the selected market during 2017-18. Four marketing channels have been found in male goat marketing in the study area. The major marketing cost components have been found as assembling -maintenance, animal raising, labour and transportation for sellers and market fee, labour and levy for buyers. Direct dealing was done between buyers and sellers and majority of goat comes in the market from outside state i.e. Rajasthan. Buyers purchase according their need and some time marketed to Mumbai market also. The gross market margin has been found lowest in the Farmer – Farmer channel. Therefore, this channel has turned out to be most efficient. It has also been found that as the number of intermediaries between producer and ultimate buyer increases, the producer's share goes on decreasing. The study has suggested streamlining of the margins of traders and market fee, price fixation based on well-defined parameters.

Table 2: Comparative Economics of Goat breeds per Goat (in INR)

S.N.	Particulars	Surati Bread				Local Bread			
		Small	**Medium**	**Large**	**Overall**	**Small**	**Medium**	**Large**	**Overall**
A.	Expenditure								
a.	Variable cost								
1.	Value of existing stock	2210.80 (40.04)	2235.98 (45.33)	2128.59 (46.47)	2186.85 (45.19)	1903.13 (40.44)	1931.84 (47.35)	1860.24 (48.27)	1907.79 (45.41)
2.	Cost of Feed	720.00 (13.04)	711.92 (14.43)	681.10 (14.87)	699.37 (14.45)	553.00 (11.75)	472.58 (11.58)	481.43 (12.49)	496.72 (11.82)
3.	Cost of Family labour	1675.00 (30.33)	1135.50 (23.02)	877.91 (19.17)	1078.18 (22.28)	1473.82 (31.32)	960.54 (23.54)	764.43 (19.84)	1057.69 (25.17)
4.	Cost of Hired labour	50.00 (0.91)	53.66 (1.09)	34.88 (0.76)	45.14 (0.93)	32.95 (0.70)	38.87 (0.95)	19.89 (0.52)	32.96 (0.78)
5.	Veterinary expenses	72.50 (1.31)	44.12 (0.89)	28.19 (0.62)	40.07 (0.83)	57.73 (1.23)	37.00 (0.91)	26.52 (0.69)	40.35 (0.96)
6.	Miscellaneous cost &	117.50 (2.13)	88.35 (1.79)	52.61 (1.15)	75.79 (1.57)	106.77 (2.27)	68.78 (1.69)	45.08 (1.17)	73.90 (1.76)
7.	Interest @ 12 % year	575.50 (10.42)	505.90 (10.26)	452.21 (9.87)	489.63 (10.12)	491.33 (10.44)	416.49 (10.21)	381.32 (9.89)	429.17 (10.21)
Total Variable cost		5421.30 (98.18)	4775.43 (96.81)	4255.48 (92.90)	4615.04 (95.36)	4618.73 (98.14)	3926.10 (96.23)	3578.92 (92.87)	4038.58 (96.12)

S.N.	Particulars	Surati Bread				Local Bread			
		Small	Medium	Large	Overall	Small	Medium	Large	Overall
b.	Fixed cost								
1.	*Depreciation*	89.70 (1.62)	140.35 (2.85)	290.35 (6.34)	200.31 (4.14)	78.19 (1.66)	137.49 (3.37)	245.50 (6.37)	145.51 (3.46)
2.	*Interest on fixed capital*	10.76 (0.19)	16.84 (0.34)	34.84 (0.76)	24.04 (0.50)	9.38 (0.20)	16.50 (0.40)	29.46 (0.76)	17.46 (0.42)
Total Fixed cost		100.46 (1.82)	157.19 (3.19)	325.19 (7.10)	224.35 (4.64)	87.57 (1.86)	153.99 (3.77)	274.96 (7.13)	162.97 (3.88)
Total Cost		5521.76 (100.00)	4932.62 (100.00)	4580.67 (100.00)	4839.38 (100.00)	4706.30 (100.00)	4080.09 (100.00)	3853.88 (100.00)	4201.55 (100.00)
B.	***Income***								
1.	Value of existing stock	2763.50	2981.30	3040.84	2985.16	2378.91	2575.79	2657.49	7603.61
2.	Sale of Animal	3999.00	3410.08	3518.02	3516.32	3573.95	3461.23	3784.21	3565.09
3.	Sale of milk	3422.40	3674.76	3337.67	3503.08	2580.23	2339.72	2046.93	2339.94
4.	Sale of manure	312.00	286.18	376.74	328.07	357.39	301.06	363.74	330.71
5.	Gross total Return per goat	7733.40	7371.02	7232.44	7347.47	6511.57	6102.00	6194.88	6235.75
6.	Net Return per goat	2211.64	2438.40	2651.77	2508.08	1805.27	2021.91	2341.00	2034.19

Marketing Channels

The five main marketing channels for transacting the male goats in the study area were:

i. Farmer – Farmer
ii. Farmer – Butcher
iii. Farmer – Local Trader – Butcher
iv. Farmer – Distant Trader – Farmer

Channel-wise distribution of 156 male goats shows 80% of male goat sold through channel II and 5% respondent use channel III and 10% farmers use channel- I. only 2-3 % respondents use channel IV.

Marketing Costs, Market Margins & Price Spread Analysis

Price spread analysis was carried out for each channel separately for both the breeds of goats and is presented in Table 3.

Through Channel I, having transaction of only local goat, the producer farmer got a higher share of 95.89 per cent in the buyer's rupee.

Table 3: Marketing Costs, margins & Price Spread in Goat marketing (in /goat)

Particulars	**Channel I**	**Channel II**	**Channel III**	**Channel IV**	**Average**
1. Net price received by producer	3962.40	3594.50	2448.06	2748.06	3188.26
% Share	95.89	94.45	80.04	81.44	87.96
2. Cost incurred by producer	67.65	79.60	0.00	0.00	73.63
% Share	1.64	2.09	0.00	0.00	0.93
3. Local trader/distant trader's purchase price	-	-	2448.06	2748.06	2598.06
4. Cost incurred by local trader/ distant trader	-	-	159.63	149.97	154.80
% Share	-	-	5.22	4.44	2.42
5. Local trader/distant trader's net margin	-	-	291.63	341.13	316.38
% Share	-	-	9.53	10.11	9.82
6. Farmer/butcher buyer's purchase price	4030.05	3674.10	2899.32	3239.16	3460.66
7. Cost incurred by farmer/butcher buyer	102.12	131.58	159.27	134.97	131.99
% Share	2.47	3.46	5.21	4.00	3.78
8. Effective Price of farmer/butcher buyer (6+7)	4132.17	3805.68	3058.59	3374.13	3592.64
	100.00	100.00	100.00	100.00	100.00
9.Gross market margin (8 – 1)	169.77	211.18	610.53	626.07	404.39
% Share	4.11	5.55	19.96	18.56	12.04
10. Marketing efficiency (Ratio)	23.34	17.02	15.37	20.36	19.02

The gross market margin was 4.86 per cent and the marketing efficiency was 16.05. It was noted that the prices of goat were fixed through mutual bargaining. Farmer sellers/buyers were often cheated by the clever traders who were able to fix the price in their favour. However, producer's share in ultimate buyer's rupee in the Farmer – Farmer channel appeared to be more than that reported by Pandit & Dhaka,2005 and Kumar,2007. According to him, the producer's share in buyer's rupee in Producer – Consumer channel of goat markets in Bihar & Bengal ranged from 77 to 93 per cent, whereas according to the present study, the producer got more than 81-95 per cent share in the buyer's rupee. The most marketing efficient channel was channel- I and channel- II.

Sustainable Farmers Income Through Goat Farming

The relative contribution of various income sources are shown in table 4.The contribution of agriculture (agriculture and livestock's) amounted to 68.70 percent of total income. Total livestock contributes 23 percent of total income out of which goat contributes 15.27 percent. The finding provides that for efficient utilization of resources, goat farming is profitable entity and it might be sustain the farmer's income over long time.

Table 4: Summary of goat keeper's income analysis

Income source	Percent contribution
A. Net crop income	45.70
B. Livestock income	
1. Goat	15.27
2. cattle	7.73
Sub total	23.00
C. Net farm income(A+B)	68.70
D. Off farm income	31.30
E. Total household income	100.00

Constraints in Goat Farming

The major constraints encountered in goat production system in the study area are listed in Table 5. The major limiting factors encountered are shortage of capital, high mortality rate, poor foundation stock, and low profit in order of importance. More than half (67%) of the respondents complained of financial problem. The availability of institutional credit was relatively easy for large goat farmers, but was a major constraint for the small farmers. High mortality and disease outbreak was a major constraint for 61% of the farmers. Mortality and morbidity losses due to diseases in goats have been a major constraint in the traditional flocks. Difficulty in getting good quality breeding animals was also a major (31%) constraint. Space is also a problem in rainy season.

Another major constraint was realization of low prices (53%) for the surplus live goats. The trade of live goats, which is unorganized and is in the hands of large number of middlemen, traders and butchers.

Table 5: Production and marketing constraints of goat farmers

Production Constraints	No of Respondents	Percentage
Financial Constraints	120	66.67
Disease outbreak & Mortality	110	61.11
Poor foundation stock	56	31.11
Lower profit	87	48.33
Problem of Grazing	30	16.67
Inadequate knowledge of management practice	60	33.33
Problem of space	45	25.00
Problem of marketing of goat	112	62.22
Low prices	96	53.33

Conclusions and Suggestions

It can be concluded that goat farming with improved breed of prevalent species and larger herd size is highly remunerative enterprise. Further it was observed the surati goat keepers followed better feeding and management practices as compared to their counterpart maintaining local goat breeds. This in turn enhanced their profit by way of higher productivity. On the basis of this study it can be suggested/recommended that local goat keepers should keep improved breed of goats with good management practices, so that the economic position of goat keepers can be improved to a considerable extent. The animal markets should be regulated similar to foodgrain markets for the smooth and effective marketing of animals.

References

Bhatia, J., Pandey, K. and Suhag, K.S.(2005). Economic analysis of sheep and goat rearing in rainfed region of Haryana. Indian Journal of Animal Sciences, 75 (12), 1423-1432.

Chandra, S. (2002). Anticipating a spurt in international trade, Hindu Survey of Agriculture, 51-156.

Dixit, A.K. & Shukla, B.D. (1995). Efficiency of different marketing channels for goats in Etawah district of Uttar Pradesh. Indian Journal of AgriculturalEconomics, 50(3), 331.

Govt. of Gujarat (2021-22). Bulletin of Animal Husbandry and Dairying Statistics. Directorate of Animal Husbandry, Govt. of Gujarat.

Kumar, S. (2007).Commercial goat farming in India: An emerging agri-business opportunity. Agricultural Economics Research Review, 20 (Conference Issue) , 503-520

Kumar, S. and Singh, S. (1999). Marketing of goat and goat meat in tribal area of Chotanagpur Plateau, India. The Bihar Journal of Agricultural Marketing, VII(4), 433-439.

Palanichamy, V., Selvakumar, K. N., Prabu, M. and Saravana , P.S. (2007). Equitable income generation through small ruminant farming: A case study in Tamil Nadu. Indian J. Small Ruminants, 13 (2), 186-191.

Pandit, A. and Dhaka, J.P.(2005). Efficiency of male goat markets in the central alluvial plains of West Bengal. Agricultural Economics Research Review, 18 (2), 197-208.

Shukla, B.D., Dixit, R.S. and Dixit, A.K. (1996). Factors influencing the sale price of goats: An economic analysis. Indian Journal of Agricultural Marketing, 10(2), 106-107.

Singh, R.S. and Hussain, T. (1996). Marketing of goat in Rajouri district of Jammu and Kashmir. Indian Journal of Agricultural Marketing,10(2),107.

Singh, S.P., Singh, A. K. and Prasad, R. (2011). Economics of goat farming in Agra District of Uttar Pradesh. Indian Res. J. Ext. Edu, 11 (3), 37-40.

Tyagi, K.K., Patel, M.D., Sorathiya, L.M. and Fulsoundar, A.B. (2013). Lactation performance of Surti goats under field conditions. Indian Journal of Animal Sciences, 83 (2), 97-100.

19

Natural Goat Farming in Karnataka

C. Shivakumara[1]., B.S. Reddy[2]., A.K. Dixit[3] and S. Kiran[4]

[1]Govt. First Grade College, Sringeri, Karnataka-577139
[2]University of Agricultural sciences, Raichur, Karnataka
[3]ICAR- Central Institute for Research on Goat, Mathura, Uttr Pradesh
[4]University of Agricultural Sciences, Bengaluru, Karnataka

In India, agriculture is the primary occupation and source of income for the vast majority of the population. More than 58% of the population depends on agriculture for their living. Indian agriculture has been expanding for a long time with the help of related industries like sheep, goat, cow, chicken, and egg production. The world's largest livestock population resides in India. For rural residents, the livestock industry is one of the most significant sources of revenue and employment. Agriculture and livestock are highly interdependent, with agriculture providing crop waste, a primary source of feed for livestock, while livestock provide manure and draught power to agriculture. The fact is that agricultural production and livestock raising work together to fully utilise a farm. In terms of giving families in rural and urban regions nourishing food, livestock is also crucial.

Because it is so straightforward, raising sheep and goats is more popular among landless, small, and marginal farmers who rely on common grazing and forest lands for food. Some of the factors responsible for the concentration of sheep and goat rearing among these categories include low capital intensity, prolific breeding, superior chevon/mutton quality, early sexual maturity, high-quality skin, low kidding intervals, good adaptability, no religious taboo against consumption, and steady returns.

A large number of mixed rearing systems are used to raise small herd and flock sizes. The population of sheep and goats in the southern region is steadily growing, mostly because there are more keepers. In all of the locations, the following feeding management systems are used.

The extensive rearing approach entails leaving sheep and goats to graze in an open field or throughout a whole pasture for the duration of the season. The expense of food is minimal with this way of rearing. More than 80% of sheep and goats are raised using a sophisticated technique. This strategy makes it difficult to effectively graze whole grasses. Thus, it would be best if we could practise the rotational grazing strategy. Transhumance, free range, pasture, and range grazing management are all included in this system. Its foundation is low resource use and low production. grazing on terrain that is part of the public domain, such as waste land, mountains, and hills.

Semi-Intensive Rearing strategy: In some flocks with restricted pasture, this strategy combines feeding in stalls and some limited free range grazing. The level of nutrients is ideal and superior to that provided by an extensive system. Although significant raising is required, the pastures are typically fenced and under restricted grazing. Along with stall feeding, shelter at night, and three to five hours a day of grazing and browsing on pasture, it also comprises. When compared to the extensive rearing approach, the price of feed has slightly increased.

Intensive rearing method: Sheep and goats are continuously housed in a small space and fed from stalls using this technique. This approach works best with an intensive operation of a medium-sized herd of 50 to 250 heads or more focused on commercial milk production. This managerial style necessitates a significant increase in labour costs. Under this arrangement, the percentage of sheep and goats in the population is quite low. A major limiting issue in an intensive system is the poor adoption of industrial technologies. The advantage of this is that the animals can be closely watched over and controlled. In this technique, the excrement is gathered in one location and utilised as an effective fertiliser. More animals can fit in the same amount of space.

The present study's necessity, approximately 7% of the nation's sheep and goats are produced in Karnataka, one of the major sheep and goat producing states. The main source of income for small and marginal farmers is sheep and goat farming. Common property resources in general, and pastures and grazing land in particular, have enormous potential. The majority of small, marginal, and landless farmers rely on sheep and goats for their livelihood, and there are many localized, improved sheep and goat varieties available. Meat and meat products, wool, and milk are in great demand. Limited research has been done in Karnataka, nevertheless, on the production and marketing of sheep and goats.

Methodology

In Karnataka's Mandya and Mysuru districts, the study was conducted. Farmers in this region have recently changed how they raise sheep and goats because they are making good money doing so. Because of the high quality of its meat, the bandur sheep breed, which is a common breed in this area, is becoming more and more important. Farmers can benefit from raising sheep and goats. Mandya and Mysuru districts in southern Karnataka have higher populations of sheep and goats. The sample for the investigation was chosen using the random sampling technique.

Analytical Tools and Techniques Employed

The Garrett Ranking Method

The Garrett ranking technique was used to record the restrictions on the production and marketing of sheep and goats. In order to determine the problem's overall score, the farmers' responses to the potential problems were collected on a rank basis.

Garrett's ranking method converts the modification of constraint orders into numerical scores. When compared to a simple frequency distribution, this technique has the key advantage that the limitations are ranked according to respondents' priority.

Below is Garrett's algorithm for translating ranks into percent.

Per cent position= 100 (R_{ij} - 0.5) / N_j

Where

R_{ij} = rank given for i th factor (constraint) by j th individual

N_j = Number of factors (constraints) ranked by j th individual

According to the table provided by Garrett (transmutation of orders of merit into units of amount or scores), the relative position of each rank obtained from the aforementioned formula was converted into scores. For each factor, the scores of all individuals were added, and then the total number of respondents for that particular factor was divided by those scores. (constraint). The mean scores for each element were then ranked and arranged in descending order.

Constraints Opined by Sheep and Goat Farmers

Table 1 provides the rankings for the several restrictions cited by the respondent in sheep and goat rearing, together with their mean (Garrett) ratings. The lack of grazing land (74.98%) and the severity of disease (PPR, ET, and FMD infection) are, in the opinion of sheep and goat rearing producers, the two main obstacles to extended rearing. Other significant obstacles cited by respondents included the use of numerous middlemen (47.83%), a lack of water for drinking and washing animals (44.34%), inadequate shelter space (42.84%), and others.

Major challenges faced by semi-intensive farmers were a lack of manpower (72.65%), a lack of transportation (68.45%), a lack of credit (62.22%), and others. The main obstacle for farmers who raise livestock intensively is a lack of labour (78.56%), which is followed by a lack of credit (72.22%), the prevalence of disease (68.89%), and other factors.

Table 1: Constraints opined by sheep and goat farmers

Particulars	**Extensive rearing farmers**		**Semi-intensive rearing farmers**		**Intensive rearing farmers**	
	Garrett score	**Rank**	**Garrett score**	**Rank**	**Garrett score**	**Rank**
a. Lack of grazing land	74.98	I	41.78	VI	36.44	X
b. Incidence of disease	67.55	II	48.56	V	68.89	III
c. Involvement of large no. of middlemen	47.83	III	34.56	IX	41.59	IX
d. Lack of water availability	44.32	IV	48.45	XI	5.68	XV
e. In-adequate space for shelter	42.84	V	17.88	XII	3.56	XVI
f. Lack of insurance protection	37.34	VI	36.88	VIII	58.44	VI
g. Inadequate veterinary services	34.05	VII	39.53	VII	52.36	VII
h Lack of market information	28.11	VIII	31.25	X	30.24	XI
i Non-availability of feed	19.31	IX	14.24	XIII	8.66	XIV
j Plagued by wild animals	15.43	X	52.45	IV	66.34	IV
k Government subsidy	14.93	XI	9.78	XIV	62.46	V
m Lack of transportation facility	14.88	XII	68.45	II	49.88	VIII
Non-availability of credit	11.34	XIII	62.22	III	72.22	II
High Price fluctuation	7.93	XIV	6.84	XV	15.68	XIII
Labour scarcity	5.96	XV	72.65	I	78.56	I
Higher cost of lamb/kid	0.43	XVI	4.25	XVI	25.44	XII

The results are in line with the study conducted by Shivakumara et al. (2016). Proper animal management strategies, such as rotational and mob grazing of animals, sustainable pasture practices, such as permaculture, and holistic livestock management are suggested in relation to the reduction of grazing land in the research area.

Family labor, where family members can be used for the labour purpose for the management, is the greatest way to handle the labour shortage concerns in semi-intensive and intensive rearing farmers. Another option is to hire skilled sheep or goat farmers from the community and pay them a salary.

The lack of grazing pasture is the main worry for extensive rearing producers because the majority of sheep and goat farmers use this strategy. The mapping, demarcation, and implementation of policy to maintain the grazing land in the state are urgently required. Additionally, producers need to receive training on how to transition from an enormous system of sheep and goat rearing to an intensive one for producing commercial meat.

References

Anjani Kumar and Singh, D. K., 2008, Livestock production system in India determinants of livestock rearing. Indian J. Agric. Econ., 63 (4): 589-594.

Dixit, A. K. and Braj Mohan, 2014, Economics of goat production in Mathura district of Uttar Pradesh. TheIndian Journal of Small Ruminants, 20 (2): 96-98.

Shivakumara, C., Reddy, B. S., Satihal, D. G.andSuresh, S.P., 2016, Productionper formance and mortalityrateunder sheepand goatfarming in Karnataka , J. Exp. Zool. India, 19 (1): 1481-1484.

Shivakumara, C., Reddy, B. S. and Suresh, S. P.,2020,Socio-EconomicCharacteristicsandCompositionofSheep andGoat Farmingunder Extensive System of Rearing. AgriculturalScience Digest, 40 (1): 105-108.

20

Nutritional Management in Natural Goat Production

Shalini Vaswani and Vinod Kumar

Department of Animal Nutrition, C.V.Sc. & A.H., DUVASU, Mathura Uttar Pradesh

India ranks first in goat population with 148.88 million goats and 10.14% growth rate (DADF, 2019). Goat meat contributes around 37% of the total meat produced from the livestock sector in India which comes from the 42% of goat population annually (GOI, 2019). Goat has served as source of livelihood support and financial security to large section of society, especially to the resource-poor farmers. However, in the current scenario, this small ruminant farm animal has tremendous potential to be projected as the "Future Animal" for rural and urban prosperity. Rapid transformation of backyard goat farming to "commercial goat industry" is taking place in the country. The perception of goat as "poor man's cow" to "preferred livestock species" is fast changing; therefore, to meet this transformation goat rearing system is shifting gradually from extensive low input system for livelihood purposes to semi- intensive and intensive rearing system for commercial purposes in India (Ramachandran et al., 2019). Due to their higher resilience capacity to climate change and better adaptability goats play significant role in ensuring food security. Goats have traditionally been a significant asset and source of protein for rural communities inhabiting arid and semiarid regions of the world. It is an endeavour of millions of small holders who rear animals on crop residues and Common Property Resources. The small holders produce milk, meat, fibre, skin etc for the community with virtually less capital investment, resources and formal training. They are conventionally raised on grazing resources. However, these resources are gradually shrinking over the periods both in terms of quality and quantity. On the other hand, there is continuous rise in the demand of meat which led to further deterioration of available grazing resources. Although, goats are reared largely for meat, but they also have potential to be established as a dairy animal. In order to turn the goat husbandry as a profitable commercial venture, it is urgently required to raise the goats on intensive feeding system because this system has potential to maintain the production statistics in regards to growing demand of goat products and transformational change in the rearing system. Although the system involves more cost and inputs, but this is justified by higher gain to farmers. Nutrition plays an essential and special role in this systems of goat farming as it has the most marked effect on production costs and accordingly on farmer incomes. Until around 80's, comparatively limited research has been carried out on goat nutrition than cattle and sheep and majority (about 45%) of research on goat nutrition, was carried out by developed countries which constitute just 5% of the world's goat herds (Morand-Fehr, 1996). But from last two decades, research on goat nutrition has been developed to obtain results that can be applied in the field, particularly in developing countries (Devendra and Mc Leroy, 1982, Galbraith, 1992).

In the present chapter, major challenges along with possible strategies for scientific nutritional management of goats are covered so as to suggest the ways to be applied at field level to enhance production performance. On the other hand, it will also give newer ideas to improve the research quality on goat nutrition and to use its results efficiently in the fie ld.

Major Challenges of Goat Husbandry

1. **Unorganized small ruminant sector:** The development of small ruminant keepers is slow due to absence of or weak social organization. They are unable to express their demands and requirements because the sector is not organised.
2. **High mortality rate:** Mortality rate of goats are high and growth rate in kids is also poor. High mortality is due to diseases like PPR, diarrhoea, pneumonia, etc. There is lack of knowledge of advance methods of goat farming, low level of prophylaxis, lack of vaccines and lower accessibility to veterinary doctors. Further, the funds allocated for veterinary services for small ruminant sector are less. Majorly small ruminants are located in remote areas and are migratory in nature; therefore the se rvices are rendered unavailable.
3. **Lack of quality Breeding stock:** Farmers are unable to identify pure breed animals because of lack of knowledge. They also face difficulty in accessing good quality breeding animals. Finest breeds (mostly males) are usually sold to slaughterers, hence leading to shortage of better quality breeds.
4. **Unavailability of inputs and services:** Usually there is unavailability of vaccines, anthelmintics, drugs and cost effective identification materials.

5. **Marketing facilities:** The market is not organized and so the goat farmers receive very low price for their animals. In addition, the availability of loans and credit is difficult for small-scale entrepreneurs as they possess limited capital for collateral security.
6. **Reduced access to credit and insurance:** Low income farmers have limited capital assets to finance their livestock enterprises for activities such as acquiring finest breeds, health care, feeding and management practices, etc. Furthermore, insurance support to livestock, a particularly small ruminant has largely been neglected by insurance providers and banks.
7. **Imbalanced feed and feeding:** Small ruminants are prevailing in local livestock systems. They are mostly reared on extensive system of rearing. They are dependent on agro industrial by-products, cereals and straws. Diets containing these feed resources are often unbalanced for main nutrients, thus is not able to meet the animal requirements.

Nutritional Approaches to Enhance Productivity

1. Feeding of Concentrate in Diet

Supplementary concentrates such as oil seed cakes, cereals and cereal by products provide readily fermentable carbohydrates, nitrogen and other essential nutrients. In most studies where concentrates were supplemented with roughage, an increase in production was reported. Shittu et al., (2011) showed that an optimal ratio of 40% roughage to 60% concentrate resulted in increased milk secretion in goats. Feeding *ad libitum* green forage with a concentrate admixture of 300 gm had a positive effect on protein conversion rate (PCR), FCR and live weight gain of dairy goats. Increased milk yield, positive effect on birth weight and growth of kids were observed (Mahfuz et al., 2018). There was also increased milk yield when dairy goats were fed 50 g of concentrate daily in addition to ad libitum roughage. It was also found that feeding green grass (roughage) alone did not meet the appetite and nutritional requirements of Black Bengal goats (Sultana et al., 2012). Gradual increase in concentrate content in goat diet also resulted in gradual increase in live weight, nitrogen balance, carcass yield and net gain (Ferdous et al., 2012).

2. Supplementation of Fats and Oils

The addition of fats in the feed is reported to increase the energy density of the feed and the feed utilization in goats. It improves palatability and reduces dustiness of the feed. However, the addition of high levels of fat in the feed, especially at concentrations above 6–7% of the dietary DM, can reduce digestion DM especially of fiber (Patra et al., 2012).

Feeding soybean or flaxseed oils 20 mL/day to lactating Anglo-Nubian goats increased total VFA, propionate and blood glucose. The significant feed utilization, may have resulted in increased milk production (Kholif et al., 2016).

Oil supplementation has been reported to affect milk composition, especially increasing the concentration of fatty acids (Chilliard et al., 2003). The study by Kholif et al. (2016) showed an increase in unsaturated fatty acids (FA) and conjugated linoleic acid (CLA) in milk, but a decrease in saturated fatty acids. An increase in CLA in goat milk was also previously found by Mir et al. (1999), when goats were supplemented with canola oil supplementation has been reported to affect milk composition, especially increasing the concentration of fatty acids (Chilliard et al., 2003). The alteration of the milk fatty acid content is because when ruminants are fed with lipid sources, they alter the fatty acid profile of the lipid which enters the intestine of the rumen (Kennelly et al., 1996). However, enrichment of essential fatty acids is also seen in other goat products such as meat. Addition of linseed oil to goat feed enriched goat meat with essential fatty acids (i.e. n-3 FA) (Urrutia et al., 2015). Significant improvement in meat characteristics of goats by adding oil in the feed (Abubakr et al., 2015). Dietary supplementation with a mixture of 80% rapeseed oil and 20% palm oil altered VFAs in the rumen and reduced the acetate: propionate ratio and methane (Adeyemi et al., 2016). Methane reduction after oil supplementation was also observed in studies by Puchala et al., (2018).

3. Inclusion of Feed Additives

Essential oils, organic acids, probiotics, prebiotics, coccidiostats, mycotoxin binders, methane inhibitors, phytogenic feed additives, etc. are some of the feed additives currently used in goat nutrition. Feeding probiotic bacteria has beneficial effects on goat health, such as, increasing average daily gain, improving nutrient digestibility coefficients, and increasing feed intake. Supplementation of probiotics in the ration of lactating goats has also shown an increase in milk yield and positive effects on milk composition such as protein content, fat yield and lactose yield (Stella et al., 2007). Inclusion of yeast cells reduce enteric methane by diverting hydrogen atoms from methanogens to acetogenic strains of rumen bacteria to increase the production of acetate (Chaucheyras-Durand et al., 2008).

However, there is a need for more research on probiotics and especially prebiotics regarding their application and utilization in different goat breeds and at different physiological stages.Plants or plant extracts and oils containing secondary metabolic compounds have been studied for their significant effects in ruminant feeding. In lactating goats, the addition of 17.6 g/kg sunflower oil, flavonoids and essential oils of Piper betle in the diet increased milk production and its composition (Purba et al., 2020). Plant oils in the ration of lactating goats improved milk fat synthesis and altered the fatty acid composition of milk without negative effects on animal performance (Bernard et al., 2008). Supplementation of garlic oil (*Alilum sativum*), Cinnamon oil (*Cinnamomum cassia*), or Ginger oil (*Zingiber officinale*) to the diet of dairy goats had advantageous effects on the milk yield and milk protein. It was also associated with the enhancement of healthy fatty acids i.e. Omega 3 and CLA in the goats' milk (Kholif et al., 2012). Feeding soybean and sunflower oil to Black Bengal goats at a concentration of 45 g/kg of the total diet had no adverse effects on nutrient digestibility and performance. However, an increase in the content of polyunsaturated FA and conjugated linoleic acids was observed in the muscle and adipose tissue of goats (Roy et al., 2013). Extracts of Garlic (*Allium sativum L.*) were found to reduce coccidial load and enhance goat performance (Worku et al., 2009). However, there is still a need to study the mode of action of these essential oils and their use in goat production.

Phytogenic feed additives have been given substantial attention because of their affordability, availability, safety, and potential antioxidant properties. The antioxidant properties of phytogenics are based on their ability to provide electrons or hydrogen ions and delocalize unpaired electrons within the phenolic aroma ring of their structure and are the central mechanisms of defence of biological molecules against oxidation (Abd El-Hack et al., 2017). *M. oleifera* has a wide range of antioxidant and anti-inflammatory polyphenols that can improve the success of reproductive events (El-Desoky et al., 2017). Supplementation of dried *Moringa oleifera* leaves at 3.0 % level exhibited stimulatory effect on the antioxidant status, reduced stress, improved seminal attributes and testosterone concentration of barbari bucks (Murlidhar, S. B. 2020).

Supplementation of antioxidants is gaining importance in animal nutrition in the context of increasing production, fertility, disease prevention, inhibiting lipid peroxidation, maintaining sensory properties and aiding in processing, transportation, storage of the feed and combating stress. Dietary herbs and synthetic antioxidants are also seen in improving feed efficiency and increasing the quality of meat (by increasing lea n meat and reduction of body internal fat in the carcass of goats (Karami et al., 2010). Antioxidants supplementation improved the meat oxidative stability in Kacang goats (Karami et al., 2011). Incorporation of different Se sources (inorganic, organic and nano) at 0.3 ppm level in diet increased plasma Se concentration, improved antioxidant, immunity, seminal attributes (improvement in progressive motility, viability, Acrosomal integrity, ROS, membrane fluidity, intracellular Ca levels, and

HOST) and reproductive hormones status. Moreover, nano Se seems to be more effective in improving fertility through enhancement of seminal attributes, antioxidant and Se status in Barbari bucks (Kumar, 2021).

4. Feeding of Forage Legume, Legume Straw and hay

Supplementing goats with feed that affluent in protein and energy is one of appealing strategies that has been carried out in developing country in order to improve production performance and boost economic benefits. Legume forages has a significant role in improving ruminant nutrition due to legume forages are rapidly degradable in the rumen which is useful to meet the requirements of rumen microorganisms for efficient degradation of low quality roughages. The feed intake, digestibility of nutrients, growth performances and carcass characteristics of ruminants' livestock that fed on low quality forages base diets and supplemented with legume forages had been improved. It was apparent that this indicated that the legume forages be used as protein supplements for ruminant livestock to improved sustainability of production Forage legumes have the added advantage of improving soil fertility by fixing nitrogen and thereby enhancing crop yield and reducing the rate of soil fertility decline. Leguminous dry fodder such as Chickpeas (*Cicer arietinum*), Pigeon Pea (*Cajanus cajan*) and Cluster bean (*Cyamous trtragoclobe*) commonlyfeed by goats is abundantly available at affordable rate particularly in rain- fed regions on account of major sown crops and not commonly feed by large ruminants.

Legume crop residues (cowpeas, peas, pulses, groundnut etc.) are relatively high in protein (about 10% or more) and, thus, they can serve as supplements of low quality roughages such as poor quality pastures and cereal crop residues. Mudgal et al. (2018) reported increased the digestibility of DM, organic matter and NFE ($P < 0.01$), intake of energy, as well as total volatile fatty acids concentration ($P < 0.01$) in the SRL in Barbari male kids supplemented with lentil straw or urea ammoniated LS in TMR.

5. Micronutrients Supplementation

Minerals supplementation was found to have significant ($P<0.05$) and positive effect on the body weight gain, nutrient intake, feed efficiency and feed conversion ratio in lambs (Kharb et al., 2017). The supplementation of mineral mixture also improved nutrient utilization, mineral bioavailability and milk production performance in dairy cows fed fodder-based diet (Sahoo et al.,

2021). Minerals also play vital role in many enzymes system and various physiological processes required for the maintenance of animal growth and reproduction as well as the health status. Sabat et al. (2022) reported that feeding of goats with green fodder and ground nut oil cake based proteinaceous diet

(12% CP) incorporated with mineral mixture @ 3% of concentrate mixture improved the nutrient utilization, growth rate and feed efficiency with higher cost efficacy. Yadav et al. (2010) found higher growth rate in goats in animals fed 150 g concentrate mixture + 10 g mineral mixture. Niaz et al. (2017) reported that goats fed 100 g concentrate mixture supplemented with 5 g of area Protein and mineral supplementation in goat diet 102 specific mineral mixture resulted higher ($P<0.05$) ADG. Dietary supplementation of Zinc from either inorganic or nano sources increased plasma Zn concentration, improved antioxidant status, immune response and seminal attributes of bucks. However, nano Zinc supplemented at 20 ppm dose considerably improved the immunity and buck fertility through enhancement of seminal attributes, antioxidant and plasma Zinc status (Singh, 2022).

6. Silage Based Feeding

Sarabi et al., 2021 studied that replacing dry forage with corn silage caused no significant effects on DMI, live body weight, milk yield microbial nitrogen, nitrogen balance, ruminal total volatile fatty acids and improved the antioxidant status in Mahabadi lactating goats. The decline in the milk urea nitrogen concentration might be related to the simultaneous availability of both energy and protein in the rumen, which led to the synthesis of microbial protein by bacteria. Hence, it was recommended that corn silage can be included in the diet of lactating goats to improve milk quality. Kumar et al., 2021 studied the effect of feeding maize silage based ration on milk yield and composition in lactating Barbari goats under intensive system and found that there was no significant difference on the milk yield and milk composition.

7. Application of Newer Feed Processing Techniques

Small ruminant feeding mainly depends on the agricultural crop residues and byproducts, low-quality hay, tree leaves, and natural grasses. However, these available feed sources are characterized by high roughage content with low protein, energy, mineral, and vitamin contents, which definitely cannot meet the maintenance requirements of goats adequately. Therefore, to enhance profitable goat production, it is necessary to determine feeding system based on feed processing methods that enables better utilization of nutrients from agricultural crop residues. Complete pellet feed prepared from total mixed ration is one of the efficient processing that ensures balanced nutrition of goats by maintaining an adequate amount of roughage and concentrate mixture. It also provides uniform feed to reduce unnecessary feed waste by increasing digestibility and palatability. Feeding of complete pellet feeding enhanced the DMI and the daily weight gain, reduced FCR that finally helps in reducing the feed cost for goat production (Ahmed et al., 2020).

8. Utilization of Unconventional Feed Ingredients

Goats feed on shrubs, bushes and trees and are natural browsers. Browsing is common in arid and semi-arid zones, as most of the browse foliages are drought resistant. Browses are considered to have high nutritional value compared to pasture grasses and crop residues. Trees and shrubs, which often represent poor quality roughage sources for cattle, because of their highly lignified stems, bitter taste and presence of antinutritional factors (ANF) such as tannins, nitrates, oxalates, sinogens, saponins, mimosine limit their utilization. But may be adequate to high in quality for goats. Tree leaves like *Melia azedarach, Morus alba* and *Leucaena* proved to be excellent feedstuffs for goats. Goats prefer tree leaves like Sesbania (Agathi, agasti), Gliricidia, Ber, Bhimal etc. Neem leaves are also palatable to goats. Goats are well adopted to tannin containing leaves, they may consume large amounts of tannins through the synthesis of tannin-binding salivary proteins, without exhibiting illness. Rumen microflora of goat contains strains of tannin tolerant bacteria. The tannins are said to bind with proteins in the rumen and lead to increased amino acid absorption at intestinal level, increase nutrient utilization and feed efficiency, thus improving growth performance. The tannins are associated with stopping bloat, impede methanogenesis and increase the concentrations of certain fatty acids such as conjugated linoleic acid in ruminant products (Patra and Saxena, 2011). The presence of phytochemicals such as condensed tannins, saponin and flavonoids in certain ethnomedicinal plants have been associated with anthelmintic activities and have role in the treatment of helminths (Matovu et al., 2020).

Inclusion of Cactus (Opuntia spp.) a commonly found shrub in arid regions, in goat feed is also gaining popularity. However, it is associated with high fiber and ash content and thus low energy and protein density, which requires specific supplementation when cactus species are used in feeding. The inclusion of cactus species in the diet had no adverse effects on the sensory properties of goat milk or on its lipid composition profile (Catunda et al., 2016)..

Feeding of Eucalyptus leaves has shown anthelminthic activity against gastrointestinal nematodes in goats (Sastya et al., 2018). Sallam et al. (2009), showed that Eucalyptus oil (*E. citriodora*) can modify rumen fermentation and has the ability to reduce methane emissions. The leaves of the trees and shrubs contain high protein content and when supplemented with other roughages the increased performance of goats is recorded.

Although the commonly used shrubs and trees are high in nutritional composition but in order to further improve the nutritional value and forage tree utilization, pelleting processing technology is also utilized. Recently mulberry (*Morus alba*) leaf pellets and *Leucaena leucocephala* leaf pellets are being prepared (Wanapat et al., 2013).

9. Utilization of Residues, Waste, Agricultural and Industrial by Products

With the increasing cost of conventional feedstuffs, many agricultural and industrial co- or by products, as well as various novel materials, continue to be evaluated as ruminant feedstuffs. Incorporation of soybean hulls, corn gluten feed or dried distillers grains, corn cobs, potato peels, vegetables, fruit by-products, industry by-products have been incorporated into the diets of livestock in reasonable amounts and have been reported to have beneficial effects on health, performance and control of feed costs. Teklebrhan et al. (2019), reported an increase in dietary protein and reduction in methane emissions when corn was replaced by corn gluten in goat feeding. Replacement of 61% of maize in the diet with dry citrus pulp and soybean hulls had no negative effect on milk yield in Murciano-Granadina goats during mid-lactation (López et al., 2014). Silages of tomato and olive oil by-products replaced oat hay at a supplementation rate of 20% and there was no effect on goat performance (Arco-Pérez et al., 2017). Marcos et al. (2020) reported that on inclusion of corn-dried distillers grains with solubles DDGS, dried citrus pulp and exhausted olive cake can replace up to 44% of the cereal grains and protein feeds in the concentrate for lactating goats. No adverse effects on nutrient utilization and rumen fermentation characteristics were observed, as well as an increase in milk yield and unsaturated FA profile of milk.

Conclusions

Although there are various nutritional program and techniques available for goat farmers to improve nutrition , increase productivity and efficiency. But, because of the different breeds unique feeding behaviours, physiological adaptation, different diet, climatic conditions, and physiological stages of goats nutritional programs of one region cannot be taken as such to other region. Hence, it is important to meet the nutritional requirements, efficient utilization of locally available resources, supplementary feeding and to enhance the profitability of farm in eco-friendly manner. Moreover, the advances in goat nutrition should be evaluated under increasing concerns of environment. Efforts are to be undertaken to facilitate the application of scientific research in the field conditions in order to transform goat husbandry into a profitable and sustainable venture.

References

A.E. Kholif O.H. M atloup T.A. M orsy M .M . AbdoA.A. Abu ElellaU.Y. AneleK.C. Swanson. 2017. Rosemary and lemongrass herbs as phytogenic feed additives to improve efficient feed utilization, manipulate rumen fermentation and elevate milk production of Damascus goats. Livestock Science. 204:39-46.

Abd El-Hack, M.E., Alagawany, M., Farag, M.R., Tiwari, R., Karthik, K., Dhama, K., Zorriehzahra, J., Adel, M., 2016. Beneficial imp acts of thy mol essential oil on health and p roduction of animals, fish and p oultry : a review. J. Essent. Oil Res. 28, 365–382.

Abubakr A, Alimon AR, Yaakub H, Abdullah N, Ivan M. Effect of feeding p alm oil by -p roducts based diets on muscle fatty acid comp osition in goats. PLoS ONE. 2015;10(3):1 -12.

Adey emi KD, Sazili AQ, Ebrahimi M , Samsudin A A, Alimon AR, Karim R, et al. Effects of blend of canola oil and palm oil on nutrient intake and digestibility , growth p erformance, rumen fermentation and fatty acids in goats. Animal science journal. 2016;87(9):1137-1147.

Ahmed, S., Rakib, R., Hemay et, A., Roy , B.K., Jahan, N. Effect of complete pellet feed on commercial goat production under the stall feeding sy stem in Bangladesh. J Adv Vet Anim Res. 2020. 7(4): 704–709.

Arco-Pérez E, Ramos-M orales DR, Y.R.L, Abecia AI, M artín-García. Nutritive evaluation and milk quality of including of tomato or olive by-products silages with sunflower oil in the diet of dairy goats. Animal Feed Science and Technology. 2017;232:57-70.

Bernard L, Shingfield KJ, Rouel J, Ferlay A, Chilliard Y. Effect of plant oils in the diet on performance and milk fatty acid composition in goats fed diets based on grass hay or maize silage. British Journal of Nutrition. 2008;101(2):213-224.

Catunda KLM, de Aguiar EM, de Góes Neto PE, da Silva JGM, M oreira JA, Do Nascimento Rangel AH, et al. Gross composition, fatty acid profile and sensory characteristics of Saanen goat milk fed with cacti varieties. Trop ical Animal Health and Production. 2016; 48(6):1253-1259.

Chauchey ras-Durand F, Walker ND, Bach A. Effects of active dry yeasts on the rumen microbial ecosystem: Past, present and future. Animal Feed Science and Technology. 2008;145(1-4):5-26.

Chilliard Y, Ferlay A, Rouel J, Lamberet G. A review of nutritional and p hy siological factors affecting goat Milk lipid synthesis and lipolysis 1. Journal of Dairy Science. 2003;86(5):1751-1770.

Devendra, C., Mc Leroy , G.B., 1982. Goat and sheep p roduction in the trop ics. In: Proceedings of the 7th International Trop ical Agricultural Series, Longman, London, 271.

El-Desoky , N.I., Hashem, N.M ., Elkomy , A., Abo-elezz, Z.R., 2017. Phy siological resp onse and semen quality of rabbit bucks supplemented with moringa leaves ethanolic extract during summer season. Animal 11, 1549–1557.

Ferdous M, Khan M, Rashid M, Kamruzzaman M. Effect of different levels of concentrate supplementation on the performance of black Bengal goat. Bangladesh Journal of Animal Science. 2012;40(1-2):40-45.

Galbraith, H., 1992. New develop ment in goat husbandry for quality fiber p roduction. Comett Un. Aberdeen, 184 pp.

KaramiM, AlimonAR, Goh YM , SaziliAQ, Ivan M, Serdang UPM, et al. Effects of dietary herbal antioxidants supplemented on feed lot growth performance and carcass composition of male goats. American Journal of Animal and Veterinary Sciences. 2010;5(1):33 -39.

Karami M, Alimon AR, Sazili AQ, Goh YM, Ivan M. Effects of dietary antioxidants on the quality, fatty acid profile, and lipid oxidation of longissimus muscle in Kacang goat with aging time. Meat Science. 2011;88(1):102-108.

Kekana, T.W., M arume, U., Muya, C.M ., Nherera-Chokuda, F.V., 2019. Lactation performance and blood metabolites in lactating dairy cows micro suppemented with Moringa oleifera leaf meal. S. Afr. J. Anim. Sci. 49, 709– 716. ht t p s://doi.org/10.4314/sajas.v49i4.12.

Kennelly JJ. The fatty acid composition of milk fat as influenced by feeding oilseeds. Animal Feed Science and Technology. 1996;60(3-4):137-152.

Kharb, R., Kumar, G, Dhama, K. and Akbar, M.L. 2017. Effect of mineral supplementation on nutrient utilization and growth performance of lambs. Journal of Exp erimental Biology and Agricultural Sciences, 5:774-779.

Kholif AE, Morsy TA, Abd El Tawab AM, Anele UY, Galyean M L. Effect of supplementing diets of Anglo-Nubian goats with soybean and flaxseed oils on Lactational performance. Journal of Agricultural and Food Chemistry. 2016;64(31):6163-6170.

Kumar, S. 2021. Effect of different sources of Selenium supplementation on performance of bucks. M .V.Sc. Thesis. Animal Nutrition. C.V.Sc &A.H., DUVASU, Mathura

Kumar R, Gupta D L, Swaroop K, A Mohd. Evaluation of silage based ration in lactating goats under stall-fed condition. 2021.36(1):36-40.

Lóp ez M C, Estellés F, M oy a VJ, Fernández C. Use of dry citrus p ulp or soy bean hulls as a rep lacement for corn grain in energy and nitrogen p artitioning, methane emissions, and milk p erformance in lactating M urciano-Granadina goats. Journal of Dairy Science. 2014;97(12):7821-7832. ht t p ://dx.doi.org/10.3168/jds.2014-8424.

Mahfuz SU, Islam M SD, Chowdhury M R, Islam S, Hasan M K, Uddin M N. Influence of concentrate supp lementation on production and reproduction performance of female black Bengal goat. Indian Journal of Animal Research. 2018;52(5):735-739.

Marcos CN, Carro M D, Fernández Yep es JE, Haro A, Romero-Huelva M, M olina-Alcaide E. Effects of agroindustrial by-product supplementation on dairy goat milk characteristics, nutrient utilization, ruminal fermentation, and methane production. Journal of Dairy Science. 2020;103(2):1472-1483.

Matovu J, Matovu H, Magala J, Tainika B. Ethno Medicinal Plants Used in the M anagement of Cattle Helminths in Kyanamukaaka SubCounty, Uganda. EAS Journal of Veterinary Medical Science. 2020;1881(3):18-26.

MirZ, Goonewardene LA, Okine E, Jaegar S, Scheer HD. Effect of feeding canola oil on constituents, conjugated linoleic acid (CLA) and long chain fatty acids in goats milk. Small Ruminant Research. 1999;33(2):137-143.

Morand-Fehr, P., 1996. Specificit′ edes sources et des besoins ′ d' information dansle secteur caprinet strategie′a adopter. ` Tintenna-Les dossiers Cirval October, 77–82.

Mudgal. V., Mehta, M.K., Rane, A.S. Lentil straw (Lens culinaris): An alternative and nutritious feed resource for kids. 2018.4(4):417-421.

Niaz, F., Sethy , K., Swain, R.K., Behera, K., Mishra, S.K., Karna, D.K. and Mishra, C. 2017. Combined effect of concentrate and area sp ecific mineral mixture sup p lementation on the performance of Ganjam goat in its native tract. The Pharma Innovation Journal, 6: 320-323.

Patra, A.K., Saxena J. Exploitation of dietary tannins to improve rumen metabolism and ruminant nutrition. Journal of the Science of Food and Agriculture. 2011;91(1):24-37.

Patra, A.K. Enteric methane mitigation technologies for ruminant livestock: A sy nthesis of current research and future directions. Environmental Monitoring and Assessment. 2012;184(4):1929-1952.

Puchala R, Leshure S, Gip son TA, Tesfai K, Fly the M D, Goetsch AL. Effects of different levels of lesp edeza and supplementation with monensin, coconut oil, or soy bean oil on ruminal methane emission by mature Boer goat wethers after different lengths of feeding. Journal of Ap p lied Animal Research. 2018;46(1):1127-1136.

Purba RAP, Yuangklang C, Paengkoum S, Paengkoum P. M ilk fatty acid comp osition, rumen microbial population and animal performance in resp onse to diets rich inlinoleic acid supplemented with Piper betle leaves in Saanen goats. Animal Production Science. 2020;

Ramachandran, N., Kumar, A., Rai, B., Singh, S.P., Kharche, S.D., Kumar, V. and Singh, R.K. 2019d. Modern elevated goat shelter with plastic slatted flooring for intensive goat production. AICRP on PET Project, ICAR-CIRG Publication. 1-6 p ages.

Roy A, Mandal GP, Patra AK. Evaluating the performance, carcass traits and conjugated linoleic acid content in muscle and adipose tissues of Black Bengal goats fed soybean oil and sunflower oil. Animal Feed Science and Technology. 2013;185(1-2):43-52.

Sahoo, B., Kumar, A., Panda, A.K., Das, L., M aradana, U., Sarangi, D.N. and Srivastava, S.K. 2021. Role of mineral mixture supplementation in enhancing productivity and profitability of periurban dairy farming. Indian Journal of Animal Nutrition. 38: 41-47.

Sallam S.M., Bueno IC., Brigide P, Godoy P., Vitti DM S., Abdalla A. Efficacy of eucaly ptus oil on in vitro ruminal fermentation and methane production. 2009;85:267-272.

Sarabi, S T., Fattah, A., Pap i, N., Mahmoudabad, S.R.E. The Effects of Rep lacing Dry Forage With Corn Silage on M ilk Yield, Composition and Fatty Acids' Profiles, Blood Metabolites, Nitrogen Balance, and Rumen Fermentation Parameters in Mahabadi Lactating Goats. 2021.p p 1-22. DOI: http s://doi.org/10.21203/rs.3.rs -1061779/v1

Sasty a S, Kumar RR, Vatsya S. In vitro and in-vivo efficacy of Eucaly ptus citriodora leaf in gastrointestinal nematodes of goats. Journal of Entomology and Zoology Studies. 2018;6(5):25-30.

Savare Bajrang Murlidhar. 2020. Effect of dietary supplementation of dried M oringa oleifera leaves on the performance of bucks. M .V.Sc. Thesis. Animal Nutrition. C.V.Sc &A.H., DUVASU, M athura.

Singh, S.P. 2022. Effect of nano Zinc supplementation on performance of bucks. M.V.Sc. Thesis. Animal Nutrition. C.V.Sc &A.H., DUVASU, Mathura.

Stella, A.V., Paratte, R., Valnegri, L., Cigalino G, Soncini G, Chevaux E, et al. Effect of administration of live Saccharomy cescerevisiae on milk production, milk composition, blood metabolites, and faecal flora in early lactating dairy goats. Small Ruminant Research. 2007;67(1):7-13.

Sultana S, Khan M J, Hassan M R, Khondoker M AM Y. Effects of concentrate supplementation on growth, rep roduction and milk y ield of Black Bengal goats (Cap ra hircus). The Bangladesh Veterinarian. 2012;29(1):7-16.

Teklebrhan, T., Wang, R., Wang, M., Wen, J.N., Wei, L, Zhang, X.M., et al. Effect of dietary corngluten inclusion on rumen fermentation, microbiota and methane emissions in goats. Animal Feed Science and Technology. 2019;259:114314.

Urrutia, O., Mendizabal, J.A., Insausti, K., Soret B, Purroy A, Arana A. Effect of linseed dietary supplementation on adipose tissue development, fattyacid composition, and lipogenic gene expression in lambs. Livestock Science. 2015;178:345-356.

Wanap at M, Kang S, Poly orach S. Development of feeding systems and strategies of supplementation to enhance rumen fermentation and ruminant production in the tropics. Journal of Animal Science and Biotechnology. 2013; 4(32):1-11.

Worku M, Franco R, Baldwin K. Efficacy of garlic as an anthelmintic in adult boer goats. Arch Biol Sci, Belgrade. 2009; 61(1):135-140.

Yadav, C.M., Khan, P.M., Panwar, P., Jeenagar, K.L., Lakhawat, S.S. and Nagar, K.C. 2010. Effect of concentrate and mineral mixture supplementation on growth performance of growing goats. Indian Journal of Small Ruminants, 16: 109-110

Index

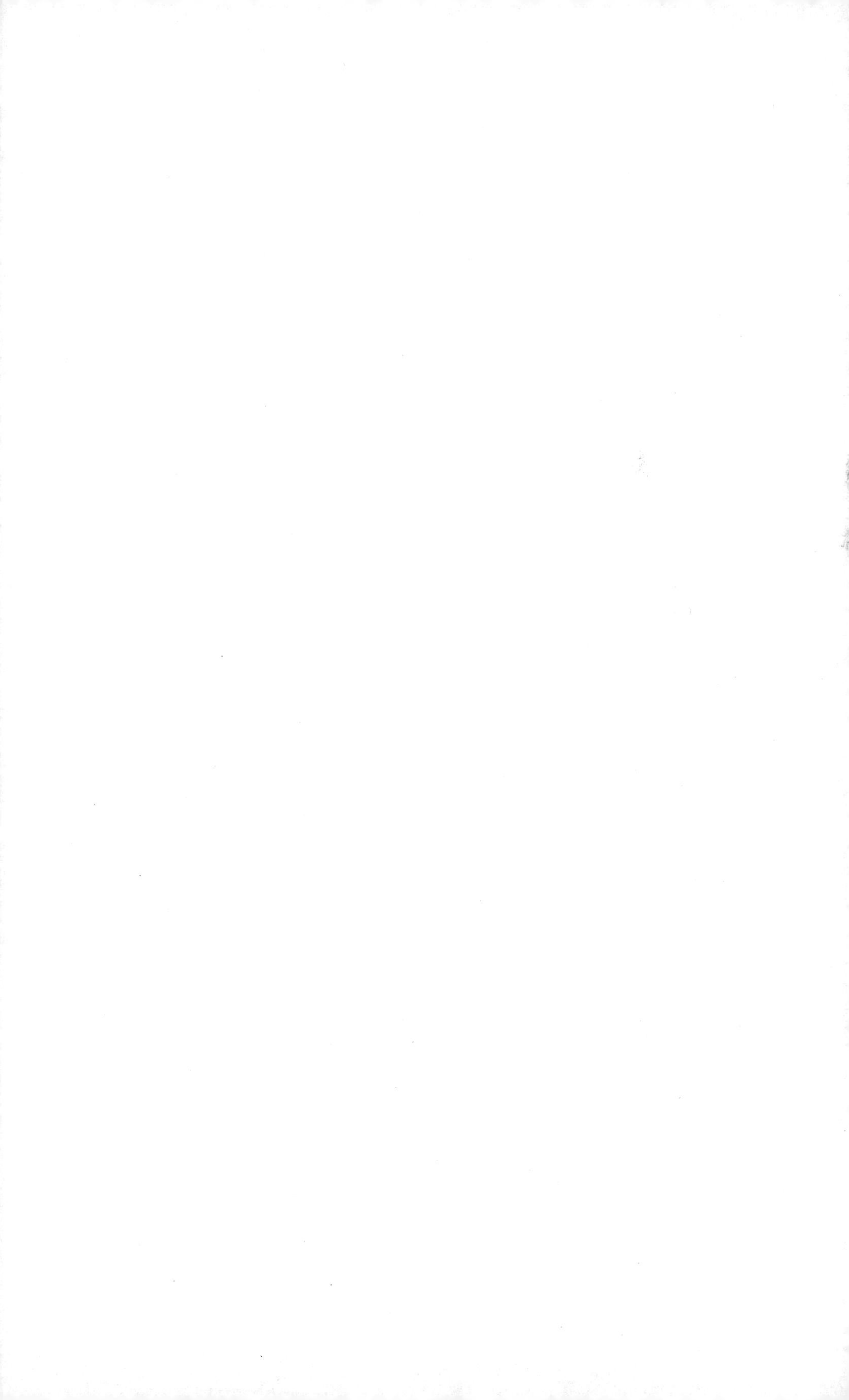